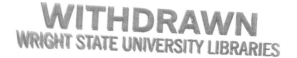
INTRODUCTION TO BRONCHOSCOPY

Bronchoscopy is one of the most commonly performed medical procedures and also defines the procedural practice of chest physicians. In most training programs, however, there is little structured education, and trainees learn by watching and doing. This book is intended as a road map for any physician looking to master or improve skills in this important area. It outlines what the authors, who are all experts in the field, think a standard approach to common procedures should be and covers everything from anatomy and equipment care to how to set up a bronchoscopy unit. Step-by-step descriptions and abundant illustrations provide the reader with detailed instructions for performing diagnostic procedures such as bronchial washing and lavage, lung biopsy, and transbronchial needle aspiration. The book also covers bronchoscopy in the intensive care unit and lung transplant patients. Advanced diagnostic bronchoscopy and basic therapeutic techniques are reviewed in the final two chapters.

Armin Ernst, MD, graduated from the University of Heidelberg and completed his residency at the University of Texas Health Sciences Center in San Antonio, Texas. He then completed his fellowship in pulmonary and critical care medicine at the combined program of Harvard Medical School. Dr. Ernst is Chief of Interventional Pulmonology and Director of the Complex Airway Center at Beth Israel Deaconess Medical Center. He is a member of multiple professional associations and has received numerous awards for his work and achievements, most recently the Pasquale Ciaglia Medal in 2007 from the American College of Chest Physicians.

Introduction to Bronchoscopy

Edited by

ARMIN ERNST

Beth Israel Deaconess Medical Center

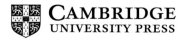

CAMBRIDGE UNIVERSITY PRESS
Cambridge, New York, Melbourne, Madrid, Cape Town, Singapore, São Paulo, Delhi

Cambridge University Press
32 Avenue of the Americas, New York, NY 10013-2473, USA

www.cambridge.org
Information on this title: www.cambridge.org/9780521711098

First published 2009

Printed in the United States of America

A catalog record for this publication is available from the British Library

Library of Congress Cataloging in Publication data

Introduction to bronchoscopy / edited by Armin Ernst.
   p. ; cm.
Includes bibliographical references and index.
ISBN 978-0-521-71109-8 (pbk.)
1. Bronchoscopy.   I. Ernst, Armin.   II. Title
[DNLM: 1. Bronchoscopy. WF 500 I618 2009]
RC734.B7I62   2009
616.2′3–dc22   2008025368

ISBN 978-0-521-76628-9 hardcover
ISBN 978-0-521-71109-8 paperback

CONTENTS

CONTRIBUTORS

Luis F. Angel, MD
Director of Interventional Pulmonology, Director of Lung Transplantation, University of Texas Health Science Center at San Antonio, San Antonio, Texas
langel@uthscsa.edu

Rabih Bechara, MD, FCCP
Director, Interventional Pulmonology Program, Emory University School of Medicine, Atlanta, Georgia
Rabih.Bechara@emoryhealthcare.org

Heinrich D. Becker, MD, FCCP
Director, Department of Interdisciplinary Endoscopy, Thoraxklinik am Universitätsklinikum Heidelberg, Germany
hdb@bronchology.org

Phillip M. Boiselle, MD
Associate Professor of Radiology, Harvard Medical School, Associate Radiologist-in-Chief of Administrative Affairs, Director, Thoracic Imaging Section, Beth Israel Deaconess Medical Center, Boston, Massachusetts
pboisell@bidmc.harvard.edu

Daniel C. Chelius, Jr., MD
Resident Physician, Bobby R. Alford Department of Otolaryngology–Head and Neck Surgery, Baylor College of Medicine, Houston, Texas

Armin Ernst, MD
Chief, Interventional Pulmonology, Division of Cardiothoracic Surgery and Interventional Pulmonology, Beth Israel Deaconess Medical Center, Associate Professor of Medicine and Surgery, Harvard Medical School, Boston, Massachusetts
aernst@bidmc.harvard.edu

David Feller-Kopman, MD
Director, Interventional Pulmonology, Associate Professor of Medicine, Johns Hopkins Hospital, Baltimore, Maryland
dfellerk@jhmi.edu

William Fischer, MD
Instructor in Medicine, Division of Pulmonary and Critical Care Medicine, Johns Hopkins Hospital, Baltimore, Maryland

Anne L. Fuhlbrigge, MD, MS
Medical Director, Lung Transplant Service, Clinical Director, Pulmonary and Critical Care Division, Brigham and Women's Hospital, Assistant Professor of Medicine, Harvard Medical School, Boston, Massachusetts
AFUHLBRIGGE@PARTNERS.ORG

Robert Garland, RRT
Technical Director, Interventional Pulmonology, Beth Israel Deaconess Medical Center, Boston, Massachusetts
rgarland@caregroup.harvard.edu

Jed A. Gorden, MD
Director, Interventional Pulmonology, Swedish Cancer Institute, Minor & James Medical, PLLC, Seattle, Washington
Jed.Gorden@minorandjames.com

Rani Kumaran, MD
Pulmonary and Critical Care Physician, The Lung Centers of Georgia, Douglasville, Georgia
kumaranrani@yahoo.com

Carla Lamb, MD, FCCP
Co-Director of Interventional Pulmonology, Department of Pulmonary and Critical Care Medicine, Lahey Clinic, Burlington, Massachusetts
Carla.R.Lamb@lahey.org

Karen S. Lee, MD
Instructor in Radiology, Harvard Medical School, Staff Radiologist, Emergency Radiology and Body MRI Sections, Beth Israel Deaconess Medical Center, Boston, Massachusetts

Deborah J. Levine, MD
Division of Pulmonary and Critical Care Medicine, University of Texas Health Science Center at San Antonio, San Antonio, Texas

William W. Lunn, MD
Vice President, Medical Affairs, Director, Interventional Pulmonary, Baylor Clinic and Hospital, Houston, Texas
wlunn@bcm.tmc.edu

Ross Morgan, MD
Consultant Respiratory Physician, Beaumont Hospital and Royal College of Surgeons in Ireland, Dublin, Ireland

John Pawlowski, MD, PhD
Director of Thoracic Anesthesia, Department of Anesthesia, Critical Care and Pain Medicine, Beth Israel Deaconess Medical Center, Boston, Massachusetts

Stephen D. Pratt, MD
Clinical Director, Obstetric Anesthesia, Director of Quality Improvement, Department of Anesthesia, Critical Care, and Pain Medicine, Beth Israel Deaconess Medical Center, Assistant Professor, Harvard Medical School, Boston, Massachusetts
spratt@bidmc.harvard.edu

Scott Shofer, MD, PhD
Director of Bronchoscopy, Durham Veterans Affairs Medical Center, Division of Pulmonary and Critical Care, Duke University Medical Center, Durham, North Carolina
scott.shofer@duke.edu

Arthur Sung, MD
Director of Interventional Pulmonology, Division of Pulmonary and Critical Care Medicine, New York Methodist Hospital, Brooklyn, New York
arthursung@aol.com

Momen M. Wahidi, MD
Director, Interventional Pulmonology, Assistant Professor of Medicine, Duke University Medical Center, Durham, North Carolina
wahid001@mc.duke.edu

Aaron B. Waxman, MD, PhD
Director, Pulmonary Vascular Disease Program, Pulmonary Critical Care Unit, Massachusetts General Hospital, Assistant Professor of Medicine, Harvard Medical School, Boston, Massachusetts
ABWAXMAN@PARTNERS.ORG

INTRODUCTION

Flexible bronchoscopy in many ways defines the procedural component of pulmonary medicine. Unfortunately, in many fellowship programs, little attention is directed toward a structured educational effort to attain the necessary skills to become a solid endoscopist. Often a "see one, do one, teach one" approach is taken, which does not lend itself to educating bronchoscopists in the best possible environment and frequently leaves little time to discuss components of the procedure at hand. Additionally, it is difficult to teach more advanced, less common procedures in this setting.

The specifics of particular procedures are rarely a matter of discussion, and neither is the maintenance of bronchoscopes. Even though pulmonologists are frequently in charge of or medically direct bronchoscopy units, the lack of this knowledge puts the new trainee in a difficult position.

It should also not come as a surprise that even basic minimally invasive procedures such as transbronchial needle aspiration are performed by only a minority of pulmonologists – reflecting the aforementioned significant shortcomings in procedural education.

In 2000, we introduced a standardized introduction to bronchoscopy for all pulmonary medicine trainees of the Harvard Medical School–associated teaching hospitals. It included a half-day of lectures, followed by hands-on training in basic techniques as well as simulation practice. It was enthusiastically embraced and quickly expanded to include Fellows from many training programs around New England. As a matter of fact, similar courses are now being introduced around the country, hopefully contributing to a better learning experience for pulmonary trainees on a larger scale. This course also provides an overview of necessary sedation guidelines and principles of bronchoscope maintenance.

This book is based on the curriculum of this course, and I am indebted to the lecturers who agreed to expand on their presentations and include them as full chapters and to all Fellows who have participated in these courses and whose feedback continues to improve this educational offering.

Armin Ernst, MD
Boston, Massachusetts

ABBREVIATIONS/ACRONYMS

2D – two-dimensional
3D – three-dimensional
ACCP – American College of Clinical Pharmacy; American College of Chest Physicians
ACLS – Advanced Cardiac Life Support
ACMI – American Cystoscope Makers, Inc.
AFB – acid-fast bacilli
AFB – autofluorescence bronchoscopy
APC – argon plasma coagulation
ASA – American Society of Anesthesiologists
ATS – American Thoracic Society

BAL – bronchoalveolar lavage
BD – balloon dilation
BIPAP – bilevel positive airway pressure
BOS – bronchiolitis obliterans syndrome
BT – brachytherapy
BTS – British Thoracic Society
BW – bronchial washing

CCD – charge-coupled device
CDSS – Continuum of Depth of Sedation Scale
CFU – colony-forming unit
CIS – carcinoma in situ
CNS – central nervous system
COX-1 – cyclooxygenase-1
CPAP – continuous positive airway pressure
CT – computed tomography
CTF – computed tomography fluoroscopy
CTZ – chemoreceptor trigger zone

DFA – direct fluorescence antibody

EBBX – endobronchial biopsy

EBUS – endobronchial ultrasound
EC – electrocoagulation
EDTA – ethylene diamine tetraacetic acid
EEG – electroencephalogram
ELISA – enzyme-linked immunosorbent assay
ENB – electromagnetic navigational bronchoscopy
EOCT – endoscopic optical coherence tomography
ERS/ATS – European Respiratory Society/American Thoracic Society
ETT – endotracheal tube
EUS-FNA – endoscopic ultrasound – fine needle aspiration (endoscope)

FB – flexible bronchoscope
FEV_1 – forced expiratory volume in 1 second
FiO_2 – fraction of inspired oxygen
FISH – fluorescence in situ hybridization

GABA – γ-aminobutyric acid
GM – galactomannan

HPD – hematoporphyrin derivative

ICU – intensive care unit
IV – intravenous, intravenously

JSB – Japan Society for Bronchology

LIP – licensed, independent practitioner
LLL – left lower lobe
LUL – left upper lobe

MDCT – multidetector computed tomography
MPAP – mean pulmonary arterial pressure

NBI – narrow band imaging
Nd:YAG – neodymium-doped yttrium aluminum garnet (laser)
NIH – National Institutes of Health
NPO – *nil per os* (nothing by mouth)
NSAID – nonsteroidal antiinflammatory drug
NSCLC – non-small cell lung cancer

OAAS – Observers Assessment of Alertness/Sedation Scale

PAD – postanesthesia discharge
PAP – pulmonary alveolar proteinosis
PAR – postanesthesia recovery
PAS – periodic acid-Schiff
pBAL – protected bronchoalveolar lavage
PCR – polymerase chain reaction
PDT – photodynamic therapy
PSB – protected specimen brush
PTX – pneumothorax

RGB – red, green, blue
RLL – right lower lobe
RML – right middle lobe
ROSE – rapid on-site evaluation
RUL – right upper lobe

SDI/DVI – serial digital interface/digital video interface
SLN – superior laryngeal branch of the vagus nerve
S-video – super video

TBB – transbronchial lung biopsy
TBBx – transbronchial lung biopsy
TBLB – transbronchial lung biopsy
TBNA – transbronchial needle aspiration
TVC – true vocal chord

UIP – usual interstitial pneumonia

VAP – ventilator-associated pneumonia

WAB – World Association for Bronchology
WCB – World Congress for Bronchology

A SHORT HISTORY OF BRONCHOSCOPY

Heinrich D. Becker

In his article titled "*Entfernung eines Knochen-stücks aus dem rechten Bronchus auf natürlichem Wege und unter Anwendung der directen Laryngoskopie*" in issue No. 38 (September 1897) of *Münchener Medicinische Wochenschrift.* O. Kollofrath, assistant to Gustav Killian at the Poliklinik of Freiburg University, Germany, in the introduction to his report on the first broncho-scopic extraction of a foreign body wrote, "*On March 30th of this year I had the honor to assist my admired principal, Herrn Prof. Killian in extrac-tion of a piece of bone from the right bronchus. This case is of such peculiarity with respect to its diagnostic and therapeutic importance that a more extensive description seems justified*" [1]. To understand this statement, one must consider the state of the art of airway inspection at that time [2].

THE PRE-ENDOSCOPIC ERA

Access to the airways in the living patient was tried already by Hippocrates (460–370 BC), who advised the introduction of a pipe into the lar-ynx of a suffocating patient. Avicenna of Bukhara (about AD 1000) used a silver pipe for the same purpose. Vesalius' observation around 1542 that the heartbeat and pulsation of the great ves-sels stopped when he opened the chest of an experimental animal but returned again after he introduced a reed into the airway and inflated the lungs by use of bellows, which mistakenly made him assume that the trachea was part of the circulating system, from which it carried the name τραχυσ ("rough" in Greek language) or *arteria aspera* ("the rough artery" in Latin) [3, 4].

Desault (1744–1795) advised nasotracheal intubation for treatment of suffocation and removal of foreign bodies. For ages, more than half of accidental inhalations of a foreign body caused the death or chronic illness of the patient because of purulent infection, abscess, fistulas, and malnutrition. Diverse instruments have been designed to remove those foreign bodies blindly from the airways via the larynx or a tracheotomy, called "bronchotomy," which was also used for treatment of subglottic stenosis such as caused by diphtheria. Also, until late into the second half of the last century, a tracheotomy also had a high mortality of up to more than 50% [5], methods were developed for blind intubation. When he presented his "Treatise on the Dis-eases of the Air Passages," Horace Green in 1846, however, was blamed by the Commission of the New York Academy of Medical Sciences as pre-senting "*. . . a monstrous assumption, ludicrously absurd, and physically impossible, . . . an anatom-ical impossibility and unwarrantable innovation in practical medicine*" and was removed from the society [6, 7], but Joseph O'Dwyer persisted and introduced the method for emergency intuba-tion of diphtheric children.

THE DEVELOPMENT OF ENDOSCOPY

Although instruments for the inspection of the body cavities such as the mouth, nose, ear, vagina, rectum, urethra, and others had been in use for ages, Porter in 1838 still stated, *"There is perhaps no kind of disease covered by greater darkness or posing more difficulties to the practitioner than those of the larynx and the trachea"* [quoted in (6)], because until then the larynx could be only insufficiently inspected by forcible depression of the tongue with a spatula, a so-called "Glossokatochon." Nobody had ever looked into the living trachea. It was only after the advent of three major inventions – (i) instruments for inspection, (ii) suitable light sources, and (iii) sufficient anesthesia – that direct inspection of the airways and visually controlled treatment became possible.

The Laryngeal Mirror

Experiments on the inspection of the larynx with the help of mirrors had been performed, among others, by Latour (1825), Senn (1829), Belloc (1837), Liston (1840), and Avery (1844), but it was not a physician but a singing teacher in London, Manuel Garcia, who in 1854 first observed his own larynx with the help of a dental mirror that he had bought from the French instrument maker Charriére in Paris [8–10]. Without knowing Garcia's work, laryngologist Ludwig Türck around the same time in 1856 in Vienna performed his first experiments with a similar device, which he borrowed from the physiologist Czermak of Budapest, when in winter the illumination was no longer sufficient for continuation of his studies (Figure 1.1). Czermak reported his findings before Türck, which resulted in a long fight over rights of priority, the so-called "Türkenkrieg" (Turks war) [11, 12].

With the use of these instruments, diagnosis and treatment of laryngeal diseases became much easier, so that G.D. Gibb in 1862 said, "It has fallen to my lot to see cases of laryngeal disease . . . that have existed for ten or twenty

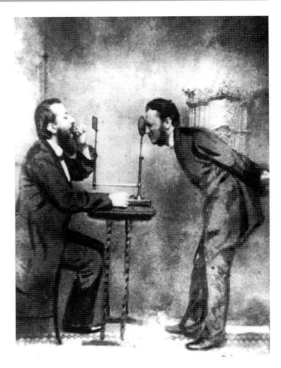

FIGURE 1.1. Czermak demonstrating the laryngeal mirror.

years, and submitted to every variety of treatment, without the slightest benefit, at the hands of some of the foremost amongst us, wherein the symptoms have depended upon a little growth attached to one or both vocal chords, which was recognized in as many seconds as the complaints had existed years. The nature of the malady thus being made out, the plan of treatment to be persued became obvious" [13]. It was also in 1862 that the German surgeon Victor von Bruns in Tübingen, with the help of this laryngoscopic mirror, could remove the first polyp from a vocal chord in his own brother. Without suitable anesthetics, the procedure needed weeks of preparation by gradual desensitization on the patient's side and much training on anatomical preparations and living larynxes of volunteers. Also his report was rejected as ". . . a daring deed that should not be imitated and the practical importance of which seems less as there would be hardly another opportunity for its repetition." One of the major problems was the indirect and reverse view of the image, which added to the difficulties [14].

The First Endoscopes and Light Sources

In contrast to other fields of endoscopy, where daylight or candlelight could be introduced for inspection of the vagina, rectum, urethra, an so on, it was only after Philipp Bozzini, a general practitioner in Frankfurt, had developed his "illuminator" in 1805 that a suitable light source for the inspection of the trachea came within sight. The still somewhat clumsy device consisted of a box containing a candle, the light of which was reflected by a hollow mirror into a "conductor," a split metallic tube that could be spread by a simple mechanism. For the inspection of organs that could not be visualized by direct inspection he used a tube with a mirror for reflection of the light and image [15].

The first suitable successor was in 1853: the instrument of Desormeaux, who also introduced the word "endoscope" for his instrument to inspect the body cavities (Figure 1.2). It was by Desormeaux' endoscope that A. Kußmaul in 1867–1868 performed the first esophagoscopies [16]. The illumination by spirit, however, was insufficient for the inspection of the stomach. The first suitable gastroscope in 1881 by von Mikulicz and Leiter was a closed optic with lenses and prisms that were electrically illuminated at the distal end by a glowing platinum wire that had to be cooled by a constant flow of water and thus was not suitable for application in the airways [17].

Esophagoscopy was performed mainly by use of hollow tubes and spatulas that were connected to proximal illumination sources. It was also the Viennese endoscope maker Leiter who in 1886 produced the first so-called panelectroscope, a tube that was connected to a handle that contained an electric bulb and a prism for illumination. The instrument was modified by many specialists, such as Gottstein, who was the first to attach a metal tube in 1891, Rosenheim, who accidentally first passed into the trachea, and Kirstein in Berlin. Kirstein

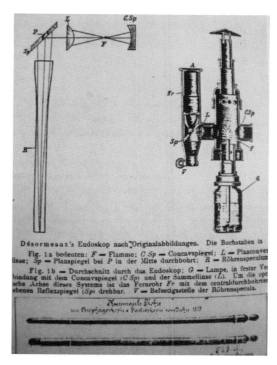

FIGURE 1.2. Desormeaux' illumination apparatus for endoscopes.

intentionally started to intubate the larynx with the esophagoscope and, after his first experience in 1894, began systematic direct inspection, which he called "autoscopy" (Greek: "αυτοσ," meaning directly without help of a mirror). "I convinced myself...that one can pass the vocal chords intentionally with a middle sized esophagoscope into the cocainized trachea and right down to the bifurcation; this experience should be eventually fructified." But as "the region of the lower trachea is a very dangerous place!...The rhythmic protrusion of its wall is...a regular and awe-inspiring phenomenon, which gives cause for utmost care in introducing rigid instruments," he did not "fructify," i.e. expand, his experiments [18]. It was the rhino-laryngologist Gustav Killian of Freiburg University who on June 4, 1895, attended Kirstein's lecture in Heidelberg at the 2nd Congress of the Society of South German Laryngologists, immediately recognized the importance of Kirstein's observation on the diagnosis and treatment of laryngotracheal diseases, and began his experiments with the new method.

In 1877 the urologist Nitze of Dresden and the instrument maker Leiter of Vienna constructed the first lens optic in which electrical illumination was performed by a glowing platinum wire at the distal end that had to be cooled by a constant flow of water when not used inside the urinary bladder, such as in von Mikulicz' first gastroscope. In 1879, T. A. Edison invented the electric bulb, which was further miniaturized by Mignon distal electric illumination to be applied to endoscopy of the airways.

The Development of Local Anesthesia

In his first report on the invention of direct bronchoscopy, Killian said, "Whether one stops inspection with the rigid tube at the bifurcation or passes on for some distance into a major bronchus does not matter for the patient. If he is sufficiently cocainized he does not even realize it" [19]. Before the discovery of cocaine, many attempts had been made to anesthetize the airways by use of potassium bromide, ammonia, belladonna, iodine solution, chloroform, morphine, and others. Nothing proved sufficient, and the patients had to be desensitized by weeks of rehearsing touching the pharynx and vocal chords by themselves before a procedure could be performed. The examiner had to be extremely skilled and swift as operations had to be performed within seconds before the view disappeared. Von Bruns suggested training on an excised larynx and on a head that had been severed from a corpse and hung from a hook before training on a volunteer ". . . who certainly could be found rather easily for a little amount of money and would suffer such not really pleasant but not at all painful or dangerous experiments" [14].

Although Morton in Boston had already introduced general anesthesia by chloroform in 1848, its use was so dangerous that it was only rarely applied in laryngoscopic operations. In 1882, a young scientist at the Pharmacological Institute of Vienna, Sigmund Freud, experimented with cocaine, a sample of which he had bought from Merck Co. [20]. He was eager to make a fortune with a breakthrough invention in science to be able to marry his fiancée. But to his later dismay his experiments in withdrawing morphine addicts from their addiction resulted in disaster. Although he had advised his colleague Koller, an eye specialist, to use a cocaine solution for pain relief when he suffered from severe conjunctivitis, he failed to recognize the importance of his observation himself that cocaine caused numbness when he put it to his tongue. Koller, however, immediately realized the importance of this observation, and after feverishly experimenting with this new "miracle drug" on rabbits and patients, inaugurated local anesthesia in his lecture on September 15, 1884, at the Annual Congress of German Ophthalmologists in Heidelberg. At the same time, the Viennese laryngologist Jellinek introduced cocaine as a local anesthetic for the inspection of the airways: "By eliminating the reflexes of the pharynx and the larynx it was possible to perform some of the operations in which even the most skillful artists in surgery had failed. The procedure completely changed. Virtuosity gave way to careful methodology, skill to exactness, and the former almost endless preparation that so often tried the patience of the physician as well as of the patient could be almost completely abandoned" [quoted in (6)]. Thus the way was paved for Gustav Killian to pursue his experiments with bronchoscopy after he had attended Kirstein's lecture in Heidelberg.

GUSTAV KILLIAN AND THE INVENTION OF BRONCHOSCOPY

Gustav Killian was born on June 2, 1860, at Mainz on the Rhine. After graduation from high school in 1878, he began to study medicine at the University of Strassburg, where one of his teachers was Adolf Kußmaul. After 1880, he continued clinical education at Freiburg, Berlin, and Heidelberg, where he passed his final

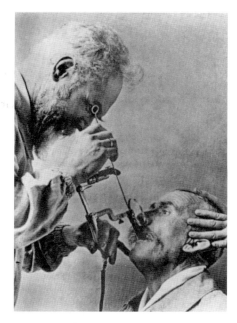
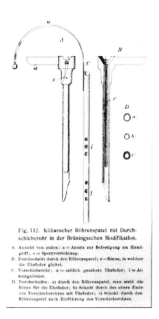

Fig. 112. Killianscher Röhrenspatel mit Durch-
schieberohr in der Brüningsschen Modifikation.

A. Ansicht von außen; a = Ansatz zur Befestigung am Hand-
griff; s = Sperrvorrichtung.
B. Durchschnitt durch den Röhrenspatel; r = Rinne, in welcher
die Uhrfeder gleitet.
C. Vorschieberohr; u = seitlich gezähnte Uhrfeder; l = At-
mungslöcher.
D. Durchschnitte: a) durch den Röhrenspatel, man sieht die
Rinne für die Uhrfeder; b) Schnitt durch das obere Ende
des Vorschieberohres mit Uhrfeder; c) Schnitt durch den
Röhrenspatel nach Einführung des Vorschieberohres.

FIGURE 1.3. G. Killian performing tracheoscopy with Kasper's electrical handle for illumination attached to his bronchoscope.

examination in 1882. Afterward he started practical work at the municipal hospital of Mannheim close to Heidelberg and later in Berlin to get an education in ENT medicine by Hartmann and Fraenkel. As he could not find employment, Killian settled down as a practitioner in Mannheim in 1887. Four months later, he left when he was asked to become head of the section of rhinolaryngology at Freiburg that was part of the large faculty of internal medicine [3, 21].

At the meeting of the Society of South German Laryngologists in Heidelberg in 1889, he gave a short report on a new technique for examination of the dorsal wall of the larynx. Killian learned about Kirstein's new technique at the meeting of the Laryngological Society in Heidelberg in 1895. Because of the experiences in Krakow of Pieniazek, who had introduced direct lower tracheoscopy via tracheostomy without any complications [22], Killian at once realized the potential of this new method of direct inspection of the trachea and in 1896 began experimental work. In tracheotomized patients, he passed the bifurcation with the "bronchoscope," a somewhat

modified esophagoscope of Rosenheim, and noticed that the bronchi were elastic and flexible; he was "stopped only when the diameter of the tube was surpassing that of the bronchi" (Figure 1.3).

After he had confirmed his findings in corpses without tracheotomies as well, he dared to perform the first direct endoscopy via the larynx in a volunteer. He noticed the flexibility of the trachea and how easily he could adjust it to the angle of the main bronchi and introduce the endoscope down to the lobar level. "I think I have made an important discovery," he noted afterwards. Bronchoscopy was born. In the same year (1897), he removed the first foreign body via the translaryngeal route on which his coworker Kollofrath reported in his paper [1].

After further experience and removal of two more foreign bodies, Killian felt safe to present his new method of "direct bronchoscopy" at the sixth meeting of the Society of South German Laryngologists in Heidelberg on May 29, 1898, and in the same year his first publication on direct bronchoscopy was printed [19]. The following years at Freiburg were full of technical improvements of the new method and the quest for more and more indications of its use. He published 34 papers concerning discovery, technique, and clinical application of his invention. In 1900, he received the award of the Wiener Klinische Wochenschrift for his paper on "Bronchoscopy and its Application in Foreign Bodies of the Lung." Because of his publications and many lectures he was famous, and Freiburg became the Mecca for bronchoscopy. Hundreds of physicians came from all over the world (the list of participants notes 437 foreign guests from all continents, more than 120 from the United States), and up to 20 training courses had to be held every year. He was invited as a popular speaker all over Europe, and patients were sent to him from as far as South America for treatment of foreign bodies, as his son, Hans Killian, a famous surgeon himself, later reported [23].

To fully understand the importance of endoscopic removal of foreign bodies, one has to consider the state of thoracic surgery in Killian's time. Most patients fell chronically ill after the aspiration of a foreign body, suffering from atelectasis, chronic pneumonia, and hemorrhage (to which half of them succumbed if untreated). Surgical procedures were restricted to pneumotomy when the bronchus was occluded by extensive solid scar tissue and the foreign body could not be reached by the bronchoscope, and it had a very high mortality rate. Lobectomy or pneumonectomy could not be performed before Brunn and Lilienthal developed the surgical techniques for lobectomy after 1910, and Nissen, Cameron Haight, and Graham introduced pneumonectomy after 1930 because techniques in safe closure of the bronchial stump were missing [24].

Thus for those who were confronted with these patients, it must have seemed like a miracle that already shortly after the introduction of bronchoscopy almost all patients could be cured. According to a statistical analysis of Killian's coworker Albrecht of 703 patients who had foreign bodies aspired during the years 1911–1921, in all but 12 cases the foreign body could

be removed bronchoscopically, although many had remained inside the airway for a considerable time; this result showed a success rate of 98.3% [25]. In light of this situation, Killian's triumphant remarks become understandable when he states, "One has to be witness when a patient who feels himself doomed to death can be saved by the simple procedure of introducing a tube with the help of a little cocaine. One must have had the experience of seeing a child that at 4pm aspirated a little stone, and that, after the stone has been bronchoscopically removed at 6pm, may happily return home at 8pm after anesthesia has faded away. Even if bronchoscopy was ten times more difficult as it really is, we would have to perform it just for having these results" [21].

Besides numerous instruments for foreign body extraction, other devices (e.g., a dilator and even the first endobronchial stent) were constructed [26]. Although the development of bronchoscopy was Killian's main interest in the years at Freiburg, he pushed ahead in other fields, too. He developed the method of submucosal resection of the septum and a new technique for the radical surgery of chronic empyema of the nasal sinuses with resection of the orbital roof and cover by an osseous flap [27]. In about 1906 he began intensive studies of the anatomy and the function of the esophageal orifice, and found the lower part of the m. cricopharyngeus to be the anatomical substrate of the upper esophageal sphincter. According to his observations, it was between this lower horizontal part and the oblique upper part of the muscle (where the muscular layer was thinnest) that Zenker's pulsion diverticulum developed. One of his scholars, Seiffert, later developed a method of endoscopic dissection of the membrane formed by the posterior wall of the diverticulum and the anterior wall of the esophagus.

In 1907 he received an invitation by the American Oto-Rhino-Laryngological Society, and it was on his triumphant journey through the United States that on July 3, 1907, he gave a lecture on these findings at the meeting of the

German Medical Society of New York. This lecture was published in *Laryngoscope* in the same year [28]. Lectures were followed by practical demonstrations of his bronchoscopic and surgical techniques and by banquets at night. On his journey he visited Washington, where he had a brief encounter with Theodore Roosevelt. In Pittsburgh he met Chevalier Jackson, then an already outstanding pioneer in esophago-bronchology at the University of Pennsylvania. He was awarded the first honorary membership in the Society of American Oto-Rhino-Laryngology and also became an honorary member of the American Medical Association and received a medal in commemoration of his visit [21].

As Killian was the most famous German laryngologist, when Fraenkel in Berlin retired in 1911 he became successor to the most important chair in rhinolaryngology. Although bronchoscopy seemed to have reached its peak, he felt that visualization of the larynx was unsatisfactory. Using Kirstein's spatula, Killian realized that inspection of the larynx was much easier while the head is in a hanging position, and he had a special laryngoscope constructed that could be fixed to a supporting construction by a hook, a technique he called "suspension-laryngoscopy" by which he could use both hands for manipulation [29]. His coworker Seiffert improved the method by using a chest rest, a technique that later was perfected by Kleinsasser and is still used for endolaryngeal microsurgery.

In 1911, Killian had been nominated Professor at the Kaiser Wilhelm Military Academy of Medicine and, as during World War I, he had to treat laryngeal injuries. He visited the front line in France, where he also met his two sons who were doing service there. After his return from this visit, he founded a center for the treatment of injuries of the larynx and the trachea. During this era he was very much concerned with plastic reconstruction of these organs, especially as he could refer to the work of Dieffenbach and Lexer, two of the most outstanding plastic surgeons of their time, who had also worked in Berlin. The

article on the injuries of the larynx would be his last scientific work before he died in 1921 from gastric cancer.

During his last years, Killian prepared several publications on the history of laryngo-tracheobronchoscopy [30]. For teaching purposes, in 1893 he had already begun illustrating his lectures by direct epidiascopic projection of the endoscopic image above the patient's head. Phantoms of the nose, the larynx, and the tracheobronchial tree were constructed according to his suggestions [31]. Because of his always cheerful mood he was called the "semper ridens" (always smiling) and, in his later years, his head being framed by a tuft of white hair, his nickname was "Santa Claus." He founded a school of laryngologists, and his pupils dominated the field of German laryngology and bronchology for years. Albrecht and Brünings published their textbook on direct endoscopy of the airways and esophagus in 1915 [25]. Like Carl von Eicken in Erlangen and Berlin and Seiffert in Heidelberg, they had become heads of the most important chairs of oto-rhino-laryngology in Germany. It was to Killian's merit that the separate disciplines of rhinolaryngology and otology were combined. When Killian died on February 24, 1921, his ideas had spread around the world. Everywhere skilled endoscopists developed new techniques, and bronchoscopy became a standard procedure in diagnosis of the airways. His work was the foundation for the new discipline of anesthesiology as well, providing the idea and instruments (laryngoscope by Macintosh) for the access to the airways and endotracheal anesthesia.

Throughout all his professional life, Gustav Killian kept on improving and inventing new instruments and looking for new applications. He applied fluoroscopy, which had been detected by K. Roentgen of Würzburg in 1895, for probing peripheral lesions and foreign bodies [32]. To establish the x-ray anatomy of the segmental bronchi, he introduced bismuth powder [34]. He drained pulmonary abscesses and instilled drugs for clearance via the bronchial route, and he even used the bronchoscope for "pleuroscopy" (thoracoscopy) and transthoracic "pneu-moscopy" when abscesses had drained externally [32]. Foreign bodies that had been in place for a long time and had been imbedded by extensive granulations were successfully extracted after treatment of the stenosis by a metallic dilator and, in case of restenosis, metallic or rubber tubes were introduced as stents. Although cancer was a comparatively rare disease (31 primary and 135 secondary cancers in 11,000 postmortems), he pointed out the importance of preoperative and postoperative bronchoscopy [34]. In 1914, he described endoluminal radiotherapy with mesothorium in cancer of the larynx [35], and in the textbook published in 1915 by his coworkers Albrecht und Brünings, we find the first description of successful curation of a tracheal carcinoma after endoluminal brachy-radiotherapy [25]. By taking special interest in teaching his students and assistants to maintain high standards in quality management by constantly analyzing the results of their work and always keeping in mind that he was standing on the shoulders of excellent pioneers, he kept up the tradition of the most excellent scientists in his profession like Billroth, of Vienna. In his inaugural lecture in Berlin on November 2, 1911, he pointed out that it was internal medicine from which the art spread to the other faculties, that patience and empathy should be the main features of a physician, and that one must persist in following one's dreams because "to live means to fight." He ignited the flame of enthusiasm in hundreds of his contemporaries, who spread the technique to other specialties thus founding the roots of contemporary inter-ventional procedures like microsurgery of the larynx (Kleinsasser) and intubation anesthesia (Macintosh, Melzer, and Kuhn).

RIGID BRONCHOSCOPY IN THE 20TH CENTURY

Main Schools

Because of the enthusiastic activities of Killian and his assistants in teaching and spreading the new technique, hundreds of specialists all over the world learned bronchoscopy and many improvements were added to the instrument. Thus already by 1910 Killian had collected 1,116 papers on esophagoscopy (410), gastroscopy (34), and laryngotracheobronchoscopy (672) for his paper on the history of bronchoscopy and esophagoscopy [30]. It was hardly possible to fol-low all traits in every continent where, soon after the introduction by pioneers, separate schools developed.

Killian's coworkers von Eicken, Albrecht, Brünings, Seiffert, and others for decades held the chairs of all important departments in Germany. They improved Killian's instruments and intro-duced new methods such as endoscopic treat-ment of Zenker's diverticulum by Seiffert, who also developed the chest rest for laryngoscopy (1922), which was perfected by Kleinsasser to the current device for micro-laryngoscopy (1964). Unfortunately after World War II the develop-ment took separate ways until recently. In West-ern Germany, Huzly of Stuttgart was the most prominent researcher in rigid bronchoscopy. In 1961, he edited his photographic atlas of bron-choscopy [36]. Riecker introduced relaxation by curare in 1952, which was replaced with succinyl-choline by Mündnich and Hoflehner in 1953. Maassen introduced bronchography via double lumen catheter in 1956. Two companies, Storz and Wolf, became the most important instru-ment makers in Germany and introduced new technologies such as the Hopkins telescope and television cameras. E. Schiepatti of Buenos Aires wrote about transtracheal puncture of the carinal lymph nodes, and Euler reported on pulmonary and aortic angiography by transbronchial punc-ture in 1948–1949 and later on the technique of rigid transbronchial needle aspiration (TBNA) for mediastinal masses in 1955, which was fur-ther perfected by Schießle in 1962 [38].

In the United States, where A. Coolidge (on May 11, 1898) performed the first lower tracheo-bronchoscopy at Massachusetts General Hospi-tal [4], it was Chevalier Jackson in Philadel-phia (whom Killian had met on his visit to the United States in 1907) who, with his

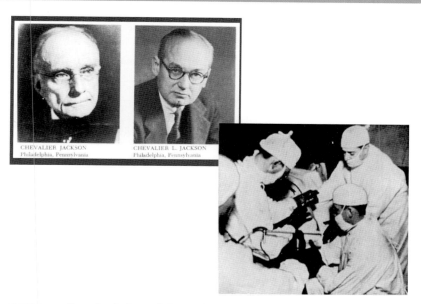

FIGURE 1.4. Chevalier Jackson, father and son, and introduction of the bronchoscope with laryngoscope.

instrument maker Pillings, made many improvements in instruments for bronchoscopy and esophagoscopy and became the "father of American bronchoesophagology" (Figure 1.4). During his training to become a laryngologist he had visited London in 1886 where he was shown the "impractical device designed by Morel Mackenzie in an effort visually to inspect the esophagus" [39]. In 1890 he constructed the first endoscope "worthy of the name" for esophagoscopy and in 1904 he constructed the first American bronchoscope. After Einhorn in New York had added an integrated light conductor and Fletcher Ingals of Chicago had introduced distal illumination to the esophagoscope, Jackson equipped his bronchoscope with a light carrier with a miniaturized electric Mignon bulb at the distal end and an additional suction channel. Confronted by many patients suffering from aspiration of foreign bodies, he invented many instruments for retrieval. In 1907 he published the first systematic textbook on bronchoesophagology, which he dedicated to Gustav Killian, the "father of bronchoscopy." In this book he addressed modern issues of quality management such as analysis and prevention of complications, rational construction of bronchoscopy suites, and arrangement of equipment and staff. Being a philanthropist, he constantly refused to have his inventions patented as he wanted them to be spread as widely as possible, and by his persistence with the government he pushed for a law for the prevention of accidents by ingestion of caustic agents. He was a perfectionist in techniques and was totally convinced that teaching had to be performed on animals before patients were treated. Therefore, he always refused to go back to England where animal rights activists prevented such training courses. In 1928, in recognition of his "conspicuous achievements in the broad field of surgical science," the Boston Surgical Society awarded him the Bigelow Medal, which was presented to him by H. Cushing "for his eminent performances and creative power by which he opened new fields of endeavor" and in acknowledgement of his "indefinable greatness of personality" [40]. He simultaneously held five chairs of laryngology at different hospitals in his hometown (Pittsburgh) and in Philadelphia. His son Ch. L. Jackson also became a laryngologist and was his successor at Temple University in Philadelphia. He was the founder of the Pan American Association of

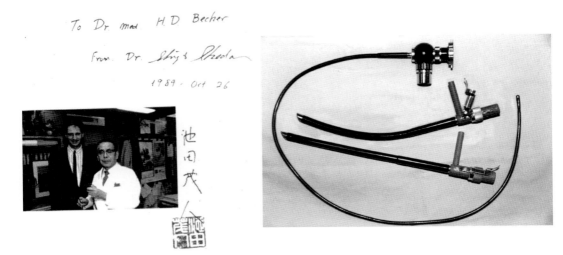

FIGURE 1.5. S. Ikeda demonstrating the first prototype of the flexible bronchofiberscope to the author. In the transition from rigid to flexible technology he introduced the fiberscope via an orotracheal tube that could be fixed in a straight position for introduction of a rigid optic and forceps if flexible biopsy was insufficient.

Otorhinolaryngology and Bronchology and of the International Bronchoesophagological Society, and was cofounder of the World Medical Association. With his father he edited the last issue of the textbook [41].

Their school extends well into our time as many of today's specialists' teachers were trained by the Jacksons, such as E. Broyles in Baltimore, who after additional training by Haslinger in Vienna introduced the telescope optic for bronchoscopy in 1940, the optical forceps in 1948, and fiber illumination for the rigid bronchoscope in 1962. His student G. Tucker became professor at Jefferson in Philadelphia, where he trained B. Marsh who keeps the tradition alive today along with Ch. M. Norris. P. Hollinger and Brubaker, who became specialists in pediatric bronchoscopy, introduced color photography in the 1940s. Hollinger's son is now a famous pediatric laryngologist. Andersen was the first to perform bronchoscopic transbronchial lung biopsy (TBLB) via the rigid bronchoscope in 1965. Sanders in 1967 introduced jet ventilation for rigid bronchoscopy.

After staying with Killian in Freiburg, it was Inokichi Kubo of Kyushu University in Fukuoka who first introduced bronchoscopy to Japan in 1907. He was joined by S. Chiba who, after training with Brünings, stayed in Tokyo from 1910. Joe Ono (who was trained by Jackson in 1934) founded the Japan Broncho-Esophagological Society in 1949. Shigeto Ikeda, who later developed the flexible fiberscope, introduced glasfiber illumination for the rigid bronchoscope in 1962 (Figure 1.5). When Ikeda, who found rigid bronchoscopy under local anesthesia in the sitting position on "Killian's chair" cumbersome, introduced the flexible bronchoscope, he used it in combination with a flexible tube that could be straightened by a locking mechanism so that he was still able to introduce the rigid optic in the same session. In the era of expanding interventional procedures, this method of combining both the rigid and the flexible endoscope today regains new attention (Figure 1.6).

Technical Developments

ILLUMINATION. After the advent of the electrical bulb, illumination became sufficient for the illumination of the airways. At first the lamps were installed separately on statives or fixed to a

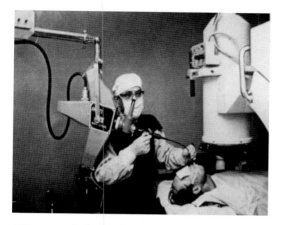

FIGURE 1.6. S. Ikeda with film camera attached to the fiberscope.

head rest from where the light was reflected into the endoscope. Connection of the light source to the endoscope improved handling considerably. Thus Killian and his coworkers preferred to use Casper's panelectroscope, in which the light bulb was integrated into the handle from where it was reflected by a prism to the endoscope, because it was not so easily soiled by secretions. Jackson, however, used distal illumination via a light guide with a Mignon bulb at its tip. By the late 1880s, von Schrötter in Vienna had developed a rigid light guide made of Plexiglas, which was improved by K. Storz, who introduced quartz. After Tyndall's first description of the optical properties of glass fibers in 1872, patents for glass fibers as a transport medium were almost simultaneously given to Baird in England (1926), Hansell in the United States (1927), and Marconi in England (1930). The first prototype of a fiberscope was presented by Lamm in Munich (1930). After Hansen in Denmark described the first fiber bundles for light transportation in 1930, van Heel in The Netherlands and O'Brian in the United States developed the first endoscopes for bronchoscopy and gastroscopy in 1953 and 1954. The rod lens and fiber-optic lighting device by Hopkins in London was adopted by K. Storz as a cold light illumination source for his rigid endoscopes in 1963. The transition to fully flexible endoscopes with image transport by glass fibers

was performed by Hirschowitz and American Cystoscope Makers, Inc (ACMI) in 1958 after Curtiss of Ann Arbor had described the first medical fiber instrument in 1955.

PHOTO-, FILM-, AND VIDEODOCUMENTATION. The first (even stereoscopic) endophotographies were performed by Czermak by use of a giant laryngeal mirror (Figure 1.1). Stein in Frankfurt used magnesia illumination for his photographic apparatus, the "heliopictor" (ca. 1875), technically the predecessor of the Polaroid Land Camera of 100 years later. Stein's camera was improved by Nitze and Kollmann. In 1907, Benda introduced color photography, which was first introduced by P. Hollinger to bronchoscopy in 1941. Soulas (1949) and Hollinger (1956) also introduced endoscopic film documentation. The first television transmission of a bronchoscopy was performed by Dubois de Monternaud in 1955. Wittmoser constructed an angulated optic for improving image transfer and produced the first video documentation in 1969.

Prospects

With the advent of the flexible bronchoscope after 1966, two developments took place: Bronchoscopy rapidly spread beyond otorhinolaryngological and specialized thoracic clinics, and the overall number of rigid bronchoscopies declined rapidly until the late 1980s and early 1990s because bronchoscopy had become much easier. Then again, the increasing number of interventional techniques demanded use of the rigid bronchoscope for safety reasons. Special rigid devices were developed by J. F. Dumon for application of the Nd:YAG (neodymium-doped yttrium aluminum garnet) laser and placement of his "dedicated stent" and by L. Freitag for his "dynamic stent." Consensus task forces of the Scientific Section of Endoscopy of the German Society for Pulmonology and of the European Respiratory Society/American Thoracic Society (ERS/ATS), as well as the American College of Clinical Pharmacy (ACCP), agreed that for many interventional procedures the bronchoscopist and staff should at least be trained in the technique of rigid bronchoscopy and should have the instrument at hand in case of an emergency. Thus in training courses all over the world, handling of the rigid instrument is taught again.

Flexible Bronchoscopy

Broad application of bronchoscopy took place only following the development of flexible instruments that could be easily introduced under local anesthesia. The pioneer of this technique was Shigeto Ikeda at the National Cancer Center Hospital in Tokyo, Japan. After Kubo and Ono had introduced rigid bronchoscopy and the related technologies to Japan, Ikeda became the proponent of bronchoscopy and pioneer in flexible bronchoscopy [42, 43]. Fiber technology had been introduced to gastrointestinal endoscopy quite some time before. Glasfiber bundles were used for illumination by cold light to replace bulbs at the tip of endoscopes, which produced considerable heat and potential damage. In addition, instruments themselves became flexible and make inspection of the organs easier. The first application was in connection with gastrocameras that had a small photographic lens system at their tip with miniature films that could be analyzed by viewing with a projector. With the reduction in fiber size and improvement of fiber arrangement, imaging via optic fiber bundles became possible, allowing real time inspection and instrumentation under visual control. However, the diameter of these instruments was too big for introduction into the airways.

Shigeto Ikeda and the Development of the Fiberscope

Shigeto Ikeda, born in 1925, decided to become a specialist in thoracic medicine after recovering from tuberculosis at the age of 23 and started his education in thoracic surgery [44]. In 1962 he joined the National Cancer Center in Tokyo where he also performed rigid bronchoscopy for diagnosis of lung cancer, using among other instruments the curette, developed by Tsuboi

[45]. For better illumination in esophagoscopy, he had fiber glass light transmission applied to the rigid optics. With regard to the flexibility of the fibers and the experiences that had been made with fiber optics in gastroenterology, he considered having the technique also applied in bronchoscopes. Thus in 1962 he approached Mr. Machida and asked for the development of a flexible bronchofiberscope with a diameter of less than 6 mm, containing approximately 15,000 glass fibers of less than 15 μm. In 1964 he obtained the first prototype of this device and, after further improvement in the summer of 1966, he was able to present the first useful instrument at a meeting in Copenhagen. The new device was reported as a sensation in the *New York Times*. After further technical improvements to enhance maneuvering and image quality (and including a biopsy channel for taking biopsies) the Machida flexible bronchoscope became commercially available in 1968, which can be considered the year of the second revolution in bronchoscopy, as bronchoscopy spread beyond specialized centers worldwide [46]. Shortly afterward in 1970 the first Olympus model was commercialized with better handling and imaging properties. In 1968 Ikeda demonstrated the new instrument at many international meetings and presented it to the National Institutes of Health (NIH) and to the Mayo Clinic in Rochester, Minnesota, where he learned about the Mayo mass screening project for early detection of lung cancer in 1970. This was the inspiration for establishing several screening projects in Japan: From 1972 to 1974 the so-called 1st Ikeda group performed a successful study on early detection of hilar-type lung cancer, including analysis of 3-day pooled sputum and bronchoscopy for localization. After the positive experience with this project, from 1975 to 1978 the 2nd Ikeda group investigated early detection of peripheral nodular lesions by x-ray screening and bronchoscopy. From 1981 to 1984 a pilot study for mass screening of individuals at risk from smoking was carried out by the 3rd Ikeda group; the results of this study led to

a big mass screening project from 1984 to 1987 supported by the Ministry of Health and Welfare, and the results of the project were published by Naruke and Kaneko.

Eager to spread the technique of flexible bronchoscopy with the fiberscope, Ikeda organized several additional groups for investigation and many training courses. In 1975 the Anti-Lung Cancer Association was founded in Japan for early detection in smokers over 40 years old. To enhance the understanding and systematic approach with the fiber bronchoscope, Ikeda developed new terminology for the bronchial tree and delicate models for training, especially in x-ray interpretation. The flexible bronchoscope was applied worldwide, and the vast majority of bronchoscopies were performed by this technique under local anesthesia. In 1978 Ikeda organized the 1st World Congress for Bronchology (WCB) in Tokyo, and in 1979 he founded the World Association for Bronchology (WAB), of which he was elected the first chairman. In 1983 the Japan Society for Bronchology (JSB) was inaugurated [47].

Ikeda never stopped improving the instrument and developing new techniques in connection with flexible bronchoscopy. His next major achievement was the introduction of a video technique, which he began investigating in 1983 and finally could commercialize in 1987. In 1979 Ikeda suffered a cerebral ischemic insult and more followed, as well as several heart infarctions, to which he finally succumbed on December 25, 2001.

In Japan several enthusiastic doctors applied flexible bronchoscopy for introduction of new techniques. Among those pioneers were Arai, performing transbronchial lung biopsies; Kato, treating early lung cancer by photodynamic therapy (PDT) [48]; and Watanabe, introducing the spigot for treatment of bronchial fistulas. With the increase of interventional procedures, the necessity for reintroduction of rigid bronchoscopy to combine with the flexible bronchoscope became obvious, and in 1998 Miyazawa

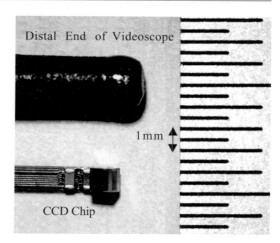

FIGURE 1.7. Tips of a regular adult video bronchoscope in comparison with a new ultrathin bronchoscope.

organized the first international conference for this purpose in Hiroshima (Figure 1.7).

Further Developments in Flexible Bronchoscopy

The ease of application and of access beyond the central airways opened vast opportunities for introduction of new optical, diagnostic, and therapeutic techniques, starting with TBLB, performed by Anderson and Zavala after Ikeda's visit to the United States. In 1974, H. Reynolds published his first experiences with bronchoalveolar lavage (BAL). D. Cortese demonstrated the potential of early lung cancer detection by fluorescence, induced by injection of hematoporphyrin derivatives (HPDs) in 1978. In the same year, K. P. Wang had started TBNA of mediastinal lymph nodes via the flexible bronchoscope, which by then was only rarely applied via rigid instruments. Also, the first endobronchial application of the Nd:YAG laser was performed by Toty in the same year, and in 1980 J. F. Dumon published his results in photoablation of stenoses by Nd:YAG laser treatment, which afterward became the most applied technique for a long time. In parallel Y. Hayata and H. Kato applied PDT after sensitization by HPD for treatment of centrally located early lung cancer. In 1979

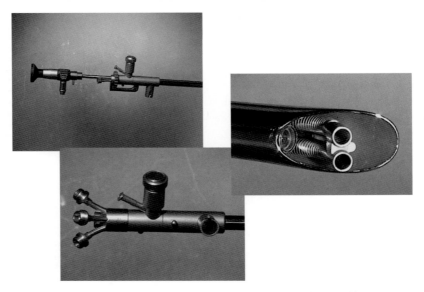

FIGURE 1.8. Modern rigid interventional bronchoscope (Dumon-Efer).

Hilarss used radioactive probes for treatment of central airway cancer for endoscopic high-dose radiation therapy. With rapid development and miniaturization of electronic imaging by charge-coupled device chips, the first video bronchoscope was developed by Ikeda in cooperation with Pentax in 1987 (Figure 1.8). Two years later, in 1990, the first dedicated stent for the airways was presented by J. F. Dumon, and in 1991 S. Lam reported on autofluorescence bronchoscopy without HPD for early detection of lung cancer. The need for local staging of these lesions was met by the introduction of endobronchial ultrasound (EBUS) in 1999 (Becker), which in addition opened a wide range of applications for diagnosis within the mediastinum and the lung and currently, in connection with TBNA by a dedicated ultrasonic bronchoscope (2003), is beginning to replace mediastinoscopy for staging of lung cancer. Early detection of lung cancer created further demand for new imaging modalities by high-power magnification videobronchoscopes and narrow band imaging for analysis of subtle vascular structures (Shibuya 2002). Endoscopic optical coherence tomography providing information of the layer structure of the bronchial wall with higher resolution than EBUS (Fujimoto 2002) is currently under investigation for bronchology. Maneuvering smart diagnostic tools inside the airways beyond the visible range has been enhanced by smart electromagnetic navigation (2003), which also supported bronchoscopic treatment of peripheral lesions by insertion of brachytherapy catheters (2005). Recently the first results of studies for treatment of asthma by thermal destruction of the bronchial muscles and of emphysema by insertion of endobronchial valves have been published (2007). The rapid growth of internet communication opened new ways for communication to enhance consulting, research, and teaching.

The exponential increase in computer capacity will create a wide range of new techniques that will also affect bronchology in the near future with regard to diagnostic and therapeutic procedures, and within the next decade bronchoscopy will gain even more importance in pulmonary medicine than it already has by now, 110 years after its invention.

REFERENCES

1. Kollofrath O. Entfernung eines Knochenstücks aus dem rechten Bronchus auf natürlichem Wege und unter Anwendung der directen *Laryngoskopie.*

MMW Munch Med Wochenschr. 1897;38:1038–1039.

2. Becker HD, Marsh BR. History of the rigid bronchoscope. In: Bolliger CT, Mathur PN, eds. *Interventional Bronchoscopy, Prog Respir Res*, Basel: Karger; 30,2–15.

3. Becker HD. Gustav Killian – a biographical sketch. *J Bronchol.* 1995;2:77–83.

4. Killian G. Zur Geschichte der bronchoskopie und ösophagoskopie. *DMW.* 1911;35:1585–1687.

5. Trousseau A, Belloc H. *Traité Pratique de la Phtisie Laryngeé.* Paris: J.B. Baillière; 1837.

6. Marsh BR. Historic development of bronchoesophagology. *Otolaryngol Head Neck Surg.* 1996;114:689–716.

7. Elsberg L. *Laryngoscopal Medicaton or the Local Treatment of the Diseases of the Throat, Larynx, and Neighboring Organs, under Sight.* New York: William Wood & Co.; 1864.

8. von Eicken C. Zur Geschichte der Endoskopie der oberen Luft- und Speisewege, v. Münchow'sche Universitätsdruckerei, Giessen, 1921.

9. Richard P. *Notice sur l'Invention du Laryngoscope ou mroirs du Larynx (Garcia's Kehlkopfspiegel du Dr. Czermak).* Paris: J. Claye; 1861.

10. Garcia M. *Beobachtungen über die Menschliche Stimme.* Vienna: W. Braunmüller; 1878.

11. Czermak J. *Physologische Untersuchungen mit Garcia's Kehlkopfspiegel.* Vienna: K. Gerold's Sohn; 1858.

12. Türck L. *Klinik der Krankheiten des Kehlkopfes und der Luftröhre nebst einer Anleitung zum Gebrauch des Kehlkopfrachenspiegels und zur Localbehandlung der Kehlkopfkrankheiten.* Vienna: W. Braunmüller; 1866.

13. Gibb GD. *The Laryngoscope: Illustrations of its Practical Application, and Description of its Mechanism.* London: J. Churchill & Sons; 1863.

14. Von Bruns V. *Die Laryngoskopie und die Laryngoskopische Chirurgie.* Tübingen: H. Laupp'sche Buchhandlung; 1865.

15. Reuter HJ, Reuter MA. *Philipp Bozzini und die Endoskopie des 19.Jh.* Stuttgart: Loennicker; 1988.

16. Kluge F. Die erstanwendung der ösophago- und gastroskopie durch A. Kußmaul und seine assistenten 1868. *Fortschr Gastroenterol Endoskope.* 1986;15:5–9.

17. Mikulicz J. *Über Gastroskopie und Ösophagoskopie.* Vienna: Urban & Schwarzenberg; 1881.

18. Kirstein A. Autoskopie des larynx und der trachea (besichtigung ohne spegel). *Berlin KliWschr.* 1895;22:476–478.

19. Killian G. Ueber directe bronchoscopie. *MMW Munch Med Wochenschr.* 1898;27:844–847.

20. Byck R. *Cocaine Papers by Sigmund Freud.* New York: Stonehill; 1974.

21. Killian H. (1958). *Gustav Killian. Sein Leben. Sein Werk.* Remscheid-Lennep: Dustri Verlag; 1958.

22. Pieniazek, Die tracheoskopie und die tracheoskopischen operationen bei tracheotomierten. *Arch Laryngol.* 1896;28:210–230.

23. Killian H. *Hinter uns Steht nur der Herrgott. Aufzeichnungen eines Chirurgen. Sub Umbra Dei.* Munich: Kindler; 1957.

24. Naef HP. *The Story of Thoracic Surgery.* Toronto: Hogrefe and Huber; 1990.

25. Brünings W, Albrecht W. *Direkte Endoskope der Luft- und Speisewege. Neue Deutsche Chirurgie Bd.16.* Stuttgart: F. Enke; 1915.

26. Killian G. Über die behandlung von fremdkörpern unter bronchialstenosen. *Zschr Ohrenheilk.* 1907;15:334–370.

27. Killian G. Description abrégée de mon operation radicale sur le sinus frontal. *Asnn Mal Oreille Larynx.* 1902;28:205–209.

28. Killian G. Über den mund der speiseröhre. *Zschr Ohrenheilk.* 1907;55:1–41.

29. Killian G. *Die Schwebelaryngoskopie und ihre Klinische Verwertung.* Berlin: Urban und Schwarzenberg; 1920.

30. Killian G. Zur geschichte der endoskopie von den ältesten zeiten bis zu bozzini. *Arch Laryngol.* 1915;29:247–393.

31. Killian G. A model for Bronchoskopy. Translation of a paper in *Archiv für Laryngologie* 13:1, Berlin 1902. Harvard, derby, 1902.

32. Killian G. *Bronchoskopie und Lungenchirurgie. Verh Verein Südd Laryngologen.* Würzburg: Stuber's Verlag; 1905.

33. Killian G. Tracheo-bronchoscopy in its diagnostic and therapeutical aspects. *Laryngoscope.* 1906;12:3–15.

34. Killian G. Die directen Methoden in den Jahren 1911 und 1912. *Semon's Internat Centralbl Laryngol Rhinol.* 1913;30:1–28.

35. Killian G. Zwei Fälle von Karzinom. *Berlin Klin Wochenschr.* 1914;7:1–3.

36. Huzly A. *Atlas der Bronchoskopie.* Stuttgart: G. Thieme; 1960.

37. Brandt HJ. *Endoskopie der Luft- und Speisewege.* Berlin: Springer; 1985.

38. Wiesner B. De entwicklung der bronchoskope und der bronchologie. Ein geschichtlicher überblick. Atemw.- Lungenkrankh. 1995;21,11;541–547.

39. Jackson C. *The life of Chevalier Jackson. An autobiography.* New York: Macmillan; 1938.

40. Cushing H. Boston Surgical Society: The presentation of the Henry Jacob Bigelow Medal. *N Engl J Med.* 1928;199:16.

41. Jackson C, Jackson CL. *Bronchoesophagology.* Philadelphia and London: W.B. Saunders Co.; 1950.

42. Ohata M. History and progress of bronchology in Japan. *JJSB.* 1998;20:539–546.

43. Miyazawa T. History of the flexible broncho-scope. In: Bolliger CT, Mathur PN (eds). *Interventional Bronchoscopy.* Prog Respir Res. Basel: Karger; 200;30:16–21.

44. Shirakawa T. The History of Bronchoscopy in Japan. Key Note Lecture, The 12th WCB&WCBE, June 18th, 2002, Boston, MA. CD edited by the WAB.

45. Tsuboi E, Ikeda S. Transbronchial biopsy smear for diagnosis of peripheral pulmonary carcinomas. *Cancer.* 1967;20:687–698.

46. Ikeda S, Yanai N. Flexible bronchofiberscope. *Kejo J Med.* 1968;17:1–16.

47. Ikeda S. The development and progress of endo-scopes in the field of bronchoesophagology. *JJSB.* 1988;39:85–96.

48. Hayata Y, Kato H, Konaka C, Ono J, Takizawa N. Haematoporphyrine derivate and laser photora-diation in the treatment of lung cancer. *Chest.* 1982;81:269–277.

49. Becker HD. The Impact of current techno-logical development on bronchoscopy. *J Japan Bronchoesophagological Soc.* 2004; 55(2)89–91.

50. Becker HD. Bronchoscopy and computer tech-nology. In: Simoff MJ, Sterman DH, Ernst A, eds. *Thoracic Endoscopy: Advances in Interventional Pulmonology.* Malden, MA: Blackwell Publishers; 2006:88–118.

2

MULTIDETECTOR COMPUTED TOMOGRAPHY IMAGING OF THE CENTRAL AIRWAYS

Karen S. Lee and Phillip M. Boiselle

INTRODUCTION

Multidetector computed tomography (MDCT) has emerged as the primary imaging modality for the assessment of the central airways. Current generation MDCT scanners can provide high-spatial-resolution images of the entire central airways in just a matter of seconds, and exceptional quality two-dimensional (2D) multiplanar and three-dimensional (3D) reformation images can be generated simply in a few minutes. MDCT imaging is particularly useful for the evaluation of airway stenoses, endobronchial neoplasms, and complex congenital airway disorders. In addition to providing exquisite anatomic detail of the tracheobronchial tree, the use of dynamic expiratory MDCT imaging can provide important functional information about the airways, including the diagnosis of tracheobronchomalacia. Furthermore, MDCT has become a pivotal imaging tool for the bronchoscopist both pre-procedurally, by helping to plan and guide bronchoscopic procedures, and postprocedurally, by providing a noninvasive imaging method for follow-up after interventions.

MULTIDETECTOR COMPUTED TOMOGRAPHY IMAGING: AXIAL, 2D MULTIPLANAR, AND 3D RECONSTRUCTION IMAGES

MDCT-acquired, high-spatial-resolution axial images provide exquisitely detailed anatomic and pathologic information about the airways. The precise size and shape of the airway lumen (Figure 2.1), as well as the presence and distribution of airway wall thickening and/or calcification, can be clearly illustrated (Figure 2.2). Conventional axial images also help to define the relationship of the airways to adjacent structures and extraluminal abnormalities not visible on bronchoscopy.

Evaluation of the airways solely with axial MDCT images, however, can be limiting and challenging. On axial MDCT images, subtle airway stenoses can escape detection, craniocaudal extent of airway disease may be underestimated, and complex airway anatomy may not be clearly defined.

Two-dimensional multiplanar reformations and 3D reconstructions can overcome the limitations of axial MDCT imaging by displaying the airways in a more anatomically meaningful representation. Multiplanar reformation images are single-voxel-thick sections that can be displayed in the coronal, sagittal, or oblique plane. Curved reformations along the axis of the airway can also be obtained, thereby allowing for multiple

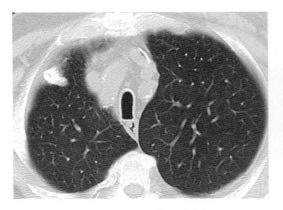

FIGURE 2.1. **Saber-sheath trachea.** Axial, noncontrast MDCT image through the intrathoracic trachea demonstrates narrowing of the airway in the transverse dimension with inward bowing of the lateral walls and widening of the airway in the anteroposterior dimension. Saber-sheath trachea is commonly associated with chronic obstructive pulmonary disease.

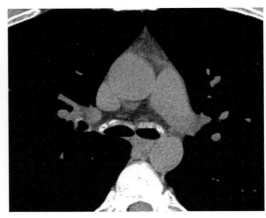

FIGURE 2.2. **Relapsing polychondritis.** Axial, noncontrast MDCT image through the main stem bronchi demonstrates smooth calcification and thickening of the anterolateral aspects of the airway wall with characteristic sparing of the posterior membranous wall.

contiguous airway segments to be simultaneously and completely imaged on a single section. Multiple adjacent thin slices can be added together to form a thick slab image or multiplanar volume reformation image, which typically varies from 5 mm to 10 mm thick. These multiplanar volume reformation images advantageously combine the high spatial resolution imaging of multiplanar reformation images with the anatomic display of thick slabs (Figure 2.3). Additionally, the use of minimal intensity projection can improve visualization of the airways within the lung parenchyma by emphasizing low-attenuation voxels. These 2D MDCT image reformation techniques allow for easier identification of airway stenosis, precise delineation of the extent of airway disease in multiple planes, and clarification of complex

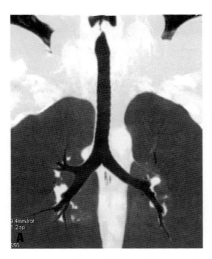
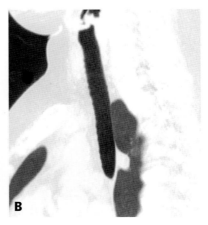

FIGURE 2.3. **Normal 2D multiplanar volume reformations of the airways.** Coronal **(A)** and sagittal **(B)** minimal intensity projection images demonstrating normal appearance of the central airways.

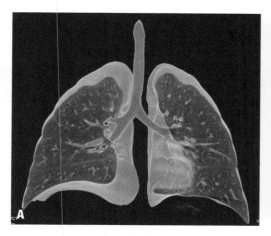
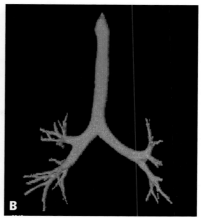

FIGURE 2.4. Normal 3D external renderings of the airways with lung parenchyma **(A)** and without lung parenchyma **(B)**. Exclusion of lung parenchyma highlights segmental bronchial anatomy.

congenital airway abnormalities. Furthermore, because these images are more visually accessible than conventional axial MDCT images, communication among the radiologist, pulmonologist, and patient can be facilitated.

Three-dimensional reconstructed images, including external and internal rendering of the airways, play an important complementary role to conventional bronchoscopy by providing detailed bronchographic and bronchoscopic road map images of the airways. External 3D rendering of the airways, or CT bronchography, displays the external surface of the airways and its

relationship to adjacent structures (Figure 2.4). These images improve conspicuity of subtle airway stenoses and enhance the display and characterization of complex congenital airway abnormalities. Internal 3D rendering of the airways, or virtual bronchoscopy, allows the viewer to navigate through the internal lumen of the airways, providing a prospective similar to conventional bronchoscopy (Figure 2.5). These virtual bronchoscopic images can provide important complementary information to bronchoscopy by assessing the airways distal to a high-grade stenosis, beyond which a conventional bronchoscope cannot pass, and by providing a unique, global, 360-degree assessment of endoluminal lesions.

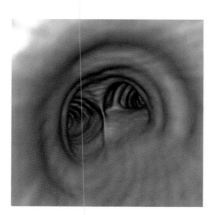

FIGURE 2.5. **Normal 3D internal rendering of the airways.** Virtual bronchoscopy image simulates conventional bronchoscopic view of the distal trachea and carina.

MULTIDETECTOR COMPUTED TOMOGRAPHY IMAGING OF CENTRAL AIRWAY PATHOLOGY

For the last few years, MDCT has increasingly become the initial diagnostic modality in the evaluation of patients suspected of having a central airway abnormality. MDCT can quickly and noninvasively determine if the tracheobronchial tree is anatomically normal, or if an extraluminal, intraluminal, or even functional abnormality of the airway is present. In the following sections,

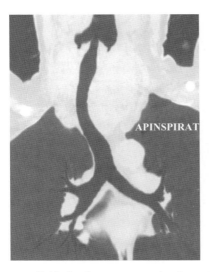

FIGURE 2.6. **Extrinsic airway compression from goiter.** Coronal 2D reformation image displays the severity and craniocaudal extent of airway narrowing involving the intrathoracic and extrathoracic trachea due to a large goiter.

the role of MDCT with 2D and 3D reformation imaging in the evaluation of airway stenoses, central airway neoplasms, and congenital airway abnormalities will be discussed, as well as the use of dynamic expiratory MDCT in the diagnosis of tracheobronchomalacia.

Airway Stenoses

MDCT-generated 2D multiplanar reformation images of the airways are crucial for accurate imaging evaluation of airway stenoses. Multiplanar volume reformation images, in particular, can highlight the presence of mild stenoses, precisely delineate the length of the airway stenoses, and identify the presence of intraluminal horizontal webs (Figure 2.6). These 2D reformation techniques not only provide important information for preprocedural planning prior to airway stent placement or surgery, but also allow for an accurate, noninvasive method of follow-up for these patients postprocedure.

In addition to 2D image reformations, both external and internal 3D renderings of the airways have been shown to be important postprocessing techniques for the complete imaging assessment of airway stenosis. As shown in a study by Remy-Jardin and colleagues, external 3D reconstructions, when compared with axial CT imaging alone, can provide important additional information about airway stenoses and allow for more accurate depiction of the length, shape, and severity of airway narrowing (Figure 2.7). In recent years, virtual bronchoscopy

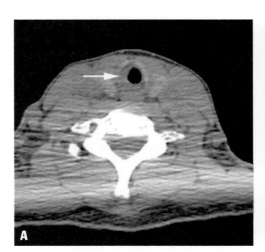

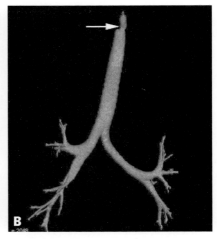

FIGURE 2.7. **Airway stenosis caused by inflammatory bowel disease. (A)** Axial, non-contrast MDCT image of the subglottic trachea demonstrates subtle narrowing of the airway (*arrow*) due to smooth soft tissue thickening along the right lateral and posterior aspects of the tracheal wall. **(B)** External 3D rendering of the central airways more clearly depicts the location and severity of subglottic tracheal stenosis (*arrow*).

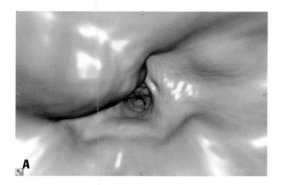

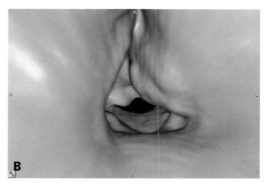

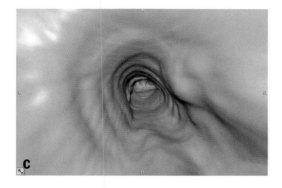

FIGURE 2.8. **Amyloidosis.** Virtual bronchoscopic images demonstrate high-grade, irregular narrowing of the proximal trachea due to amyloidosis from both proximal **(A)** and distal **(B)** perspectives. **(C)** Virtual bronchoscopic image obtained at a level distal to the stenosis shows diffuse airway abnormality with patency of the distal trachea and carina.

has become a rapidly emerging technique for the evaluation of airway stenosis, as this method provides an intraluminal perspective of the airways distal to an area of high-grade luminal narrowing, beyond where a flexible bronchoscope can pass. Furthermore, virtual bronchoscopy can depict airway stenoses from a distal viewpoint, thereby allowing for a comprehensive depiction of the airway narrowing from multiple perspectives (Figure 2.8).

MDCT imaging with 2D multiplanar and 3D reconstruction techniques has been shown to be a highly sensitive, specific, and accurate method for the detection and diagnosis of airway stenoses when compared with flexible bronchoscopy, with reported sensitivities ranging from 87% to 92% and specificities ranging from 86% to 95%. In addition, Hoppe and colleagues demonstrated that 2D sagittal reformatted images and virtual bronchoscopic images were more accurate than axial MDCT images alone in the detection of bronchoscopically confirmed central airway stenoses, with accuracies of 96.5%, 98%, and

96%, respectively. These findings underscore the added value of 2D multiplanar and 3D reconstructions in the MDCT imaging evaluation of airway narrowing.

Central Airway Neoplasms

MDCT is the imaging modality of choice for the diagnosis, staging, and preoperative planning of central airway neoplasms. The sensitivity of MDCT for identifying airway abnormalities, including neoplasms, is 97%. MDCT allows for accurate determination of the 3D size, including craniocaudal length, and precise location of the tumor within the airways. MDCT clearly maps the relationship of the airway neoplasm to surrounding airways and vasculature, providing critical preoperative information for the surgeon. The intraluminal and extraluminal extent of tumor and presence of postobstructive complications (including air trapping, mucous plugging, atelectasis, and pneumonia) are readily demonstrated on MDCT (Figure 2.9). By detecting the presence of lymphadenopathy and distant

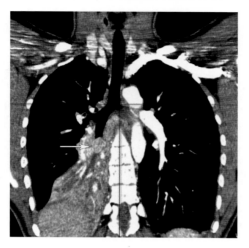

FIGURE 2.9. Endobronchial carcinoid tumor. Coronal multiplanar reformatted image shows a predominantly intraluminal, enhancing, round mass (*arrow*) obstructing the right lower lobe bronchus resulting in lobar collapse.

metastases, MDCT facilitates accurate staging of the disease and aids in guiding biopsy procedures.

MDCT imaging can determine the amenability of airway neoplasms for complete surgical resection. The approach, type, and extent of surgical resection, including the need for prosthetic airway reconstruction and adjuvant therapy, can be anticipated based on MDCT imaging findings. For those patients who are deemed to be

nonsurgical candidates, MDCT can assess the patency of the airways distal to the neoplasm and determine suitability of the airways for airway stent placement.

Although MDCT is highly sensitive for detecting the presence of central airway neoplasms, only rarely do MDCT imaging features allow for an exact diagnosis. Certain MDCT imaging characteristics, however, do enable classification of a neoplasm as benign or malignant.

Benign neoplasms typically are small in size, measuring 2 cm or less in diameter, and appear as round, polypoid, or sessile, focal intraluminal masses. These lesions are well circumscribed and smoothly marginated without evidence of mediastinal invasion or extraluminal extension.

In contrast, malignant airway neoplasms are usually larger in size, often measuring 2–4 cm in diameter. These lesions are often flat or lobulated masses, and their margins are irregular or poorly defined (Figure 2.10). Extramural extension and mediastinal invasion may be present. In 10% of malignant airway neoplasms, circumferential airway wall thickening and associated luminal narrowing may be present, findings that are highly characteristic of malignancy. Lymphadenopathy is more commonly seen in cases of malignancy; however, reactive lymphadenopathy

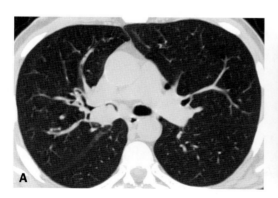

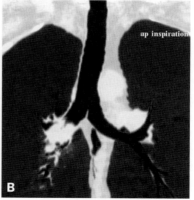

FIGURE 2.10. Squamous cell carcinoma. (A) Axial, noncontrast MDCT image demonstrates a lobulated mass with ill-defined borders within the proximal right main stem bronchus causing near complete occlusion. **(B)** Coronal minimal intensity projection image more clearly displays the size and location of this endobronchial mass with extraluminal extension.

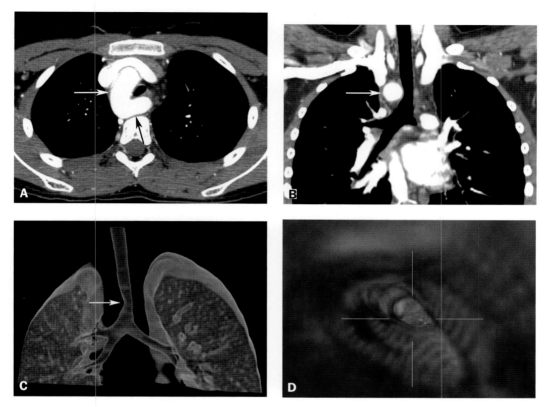

FIGURE 2.11. Right aortic arch with aberrant left subclavian artery. (A) Axial, contrast-enhanced MDCT image shows a right aortic arch (*white arrow*) with aberrant left subclavian artery (*black arrow*) coursing posteriorly to the trachea, causing airway luminal narrowing. **(B)** Coronal multiplanar reformatted image shows the origin of the aberrant left subclavian artery (*arrow*) causing extrinsic lateral compression on the trachea. External **(C)** and internal **(D)** 3D renderings of the trachea clearly depict extent and length of extrinsic airway compression and luminal narrowing (*arrow*). *Courtesy of Edward Lee, MD.*

may be present in both benign and malignant tumors that are complicated by postobstruction pneumonia. Thus, biopsy of enlarged lymph nodes is necessary for accurate staging purposes.

Although most airway neoplasms are soft tissue in attenuation (a nonspecific finding), in some cases, the MDCT density of an airway lesion can enable a specific diagnosis. MDCT is remarkably sensitive and specific in the detection of fat, and the identification of fat within an airway neoplasm indicates a benign etiology. The most common fat-containing airway tumors include lipomas and hamartomas. The presence of calcification within an airway neoplasm can be seen both in carcinoids and in cartilaginous tumors,

including chondroma, chondroblastoma, and chondrosarcoma. Recognition of both fat and calcification within an airway tumor is virtually diagnostic for a hamartoma. MDCT enhancement characteristics may also further enable a diagnosis. For example, carcinoid tumors characteristically demonstrate marked homogenous enhancement after the administration of intravenous contrast (Figure 2.9).

Congenital Airway Disorders

MDCT imaging is an excellent, noninvasive technique for evaluating congenital airway abnormalities, particularly in young children in whom fiber-optic bronchoscopy is often avoided

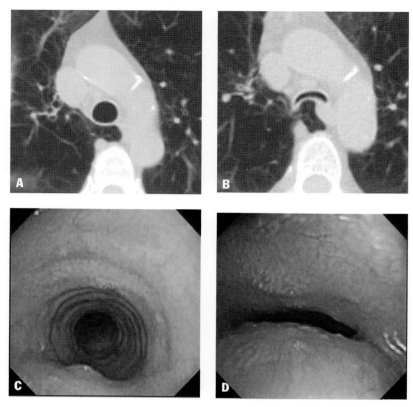

FIGURE 2.12. **Tracheomalacia. (A)** Axial, noncontrast MDCT image of the trachea at end inspiration shows normal configuration of the airway. **(B)** Axial, noncontrast MDCT image of the trachea obtained at the same level as in **(A)** but during dynamic expiration demonstrates marked collapse of the airway lumen with a "frown-like" appearance, consistent with severe malacia. Conventional bronchoscopic images on inspiration **(C)** and expiration **(D)** confirm MDCT findings.

because of its invasive nature and need for general anesthesia. Recently, Heyer and colleagues described low-dose MDCT techniques that substantially limit the radiation dose to children but remain 87% sensitive for diagnosing central airway abnormalities with a positive predictive value of 97%. MDCT can easily elucidate the cause of congenital airway stenoses, which may be due to either an intrinsic cause such as complete tracheal rings, or an extrinsic cause, such as compression resulting from vascular rings, pulmonary slings, or other aberrant or abnormal mediastinal vasculature (Figure 2.11). Congenital airway anomalies, including tracheoesophageal fistulas, tracheal and bronchial hypoplasia or agenesis, supernumerary or accessory airways, and anomalous airway branching, can be clearly illustrated, particularly with multiplanar and 3D reformation techniques.

Tracheobronchomalacia: Use of Dynamic Expiratory MDCT

Tracheobronchomalacia is a condition defined by excessive collapse of the central airways during expiration due to weakness of the airway walls and supporting cartilage. Tracheobronchomalacia is believed to be a widely underdiagnosed condition, as this disease escapes detection on routine end-inspiratory MDCT imaging.

Paired end-inspiratory, dynamic expiratory MDCT imaging of the central airways has been shown to be a highly sensitive method for

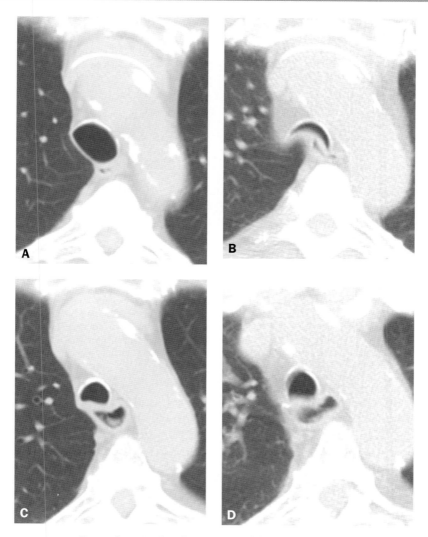

FIGURE 2.13. **Pre- and posttracheoplasty surgery.** Axial noncontrast MDCT images of the trachea at the level of the aortic arch prior to surgery at end inspiration **(A)** and during dynamic expiration **(B)** show severe collapse of the trachea consistent with tracheomalacia. Post-tracheoplasty, axial noncontrast MDCT images at end inspiration **(C)** and during dynamic expiration **(D)** demonstrate resolution of tracheomalacia.

detecting excessive airway collapse in patients with bronchoscopically proven tracheobronchomalacia. Similar to that on bronchoscopy, the diagnosis of airway malacia on MDCT is established when the cross-sectional area of the airway lumen collapses more than 50% on dynamic expiration when compared with end inspiration (Figure 2.12). Although a diagnosis of tracheobronchomalacia is usually made quantitatively,

a characteristic "frown-like" appearance of the airway caused by excessive anterior bowing of the posterior membranous airway wall may be observed in approximately half of patients with this condition (Figure 2.12B). From a practical standpoint, this sign can be helpful in identifying tracheobronchomalacia when patients inadvertently breathe during routine CT studies. Ideally, however, the diagnosis should be confirmed on a

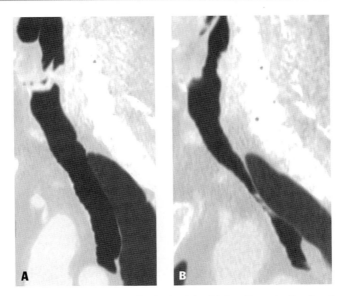

FIGURE 2.14. **Tracheomalacia. (A)** Sagittal minimal intensity projection image at end inspiration demonstrates a normal appearance of the trachea. **(B)** On dynamic expiration, sagittal minimal intensity projection image not only shows severe anteroposterior collapse of the intrathoracic trachea, but also clearly delineates the craniocaudal extent of malacia.

dedicated dynamic expiratory CT study. MDCT imaging during dynamic expiration, or forceful exhalation, is preferable to imaging at end expiration as a greater degree of collapse is elicited with the former technique in patients with airway malacia. The dynamic expiratory technique has recently been shown to have a high sensitivity (97%) for detecting tracheobronchomalacia in comparison with the "gold standard" of bronchoscopy. Thus, MDCT can be used to screen patients for this condition. Additionally, dynamic expiratory MDCT imaging allows for visualization of air trapping within the lung parenchyma, a finding that is increased in frequency and severity in patients with tracheobronchomalacia in comparison to patients without this condition. After a diagnosis of tracheobronchomalacia has been established, MDCT imaging can facilitate airway stent placement and presurgical planning for tracheoplasty, a novel technique that reinforces the posterior membranous wall with a Marlex graft (Figure 2.13). This promising treatment is reserved for patients with severely symp-

tomatic tracheobronchomalacia. Sagittal 2D reformation images along the axis of the trachea, and 3D external reconstructions are particularly useful in delineating the longitudinal extent and severity of airway collapse during dynamic expiration (Figures 2.14 and 2.15).

MULTIDETECTOR COMPUTED TOMOGRAPHY IMAGING: COMPLEMENTARY ROLE TO BRONCHOSCOPY

Although MDCT can never completely supplant conventional bronchoscopy, we emphasize that crucial supplementary information can be gleaned from MDCT imaging both preprocedurally and postprocedurally. In certain cases, MDCT may obviate the need for diagnostic bronchoscopy, thus allowing the bronchoscopist to proceed directly to a therapeutic bronchoscopic procedure. Many endobronchial procedures including laser photocoagulation, brachytherapy, endobronchial cryotherapy, and

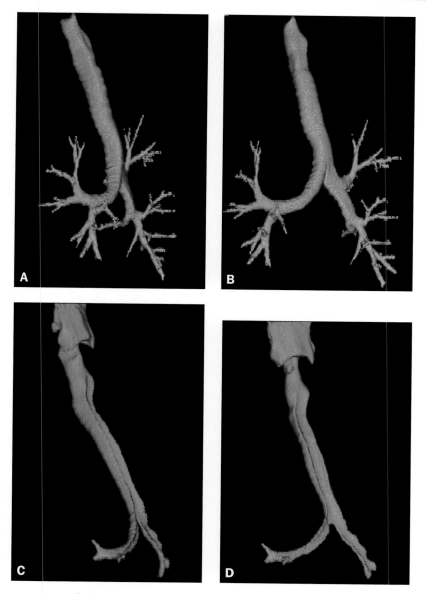

FIGURE 2.15. **Tracheobronchomalacia.** Sagittal **(A)** and oblique **(B)** 3D external reconstructions of the central airways at end inspiration demonstrate normal trachea and bronchi. Sagittal **(C)** and oblique **(D)** 3D external reconstruction images of the central airways during dynamic expiration show diffuse tracheobronchomalacia with pruned appearance of the segmental bronchi due to severe luminal collapse.

endobronchial stent placement can be facilitated with MDCT image guidance. Transbronchial biopsies, in particular, can benefit from both virtual and real-time image guidance provided by MDCT. Virtual bronchoscopy in combination with MDCT axial and 2D reformation images can help the pulmonologist determine the ideal location for transbronchial biopsy, particularly for those endobronchially invisible lesions that do not cause mucosal or airway distortion. Additionally, virtual bronchoscopy can help plan the optimal course for passage of bronchoscopic instruments into lesions lying beyond the optic limits of a conventional bronchoscope. As opposed to virtual techniques, CT fluoroscopy can provide real-time, active guidance of transbronchial biopsies. With CT fluoroscopy, the position of the needle can be easily confirmed or simply adjusted.

Prestent and Poststent Evaluation

In addition to providing both virtual and real-time guidance for transbronchial biopsies, MDCT can also provide important preprocedural and postprocedural information for endobronchial stent placement. Prior to stent placement, MDCT serves to elucidate the anatomy, pathology, severity, and extent of airway obstruction. Imaging information can help identify the source of airway obstruction as being caused by extraluminal compression, intraluminal disease, or intrinsic disease, such as from tracheobronchomalacia. Additionally, MDCT can detail distal airway anatomy not visualized with conventional bronchoscopy. Importantly, MDCT imaging findings can help decide which patients are amenable to surgical resection and which patients are candidates for palliative options such as airway stenting. For those patients suitable for endobronchial stenting, MDCT findings can help select the type, endoluminal size, and length of stent needed.

Although flexible bronchoscopy is the conventional method of follow-up after stent placement, MDCT is ideally suited to image the airways after endobronchial stenting. All endobronchial stents, whether silicone or metallic, create minimal artifacts on MDCT, and therefore are well visualized on MDCT imaging. The precise location, shape, and patency of the stent as well as its relationship to adjacent airways can be clearly delineated with MDCT and multiplanar imaging. Furthermore, MDCT is highly accurate in detecting stent complications, including malpositioning, migration, fracture, size discrepancy between stent and airway, development of excessive in-stent granulation tissue, external airway stent compression with continued

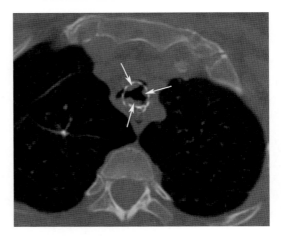

FIGURE 2.16. Size discrepancy between tracheal stent and airway lumen. Axial noncontrast MDCT image of the trachea demonstrates tracheal lumen to be larger than the caliber of the tracheal stent. Additionally, polypoid soft-tissue opacities (*arrows*) projecting into the lumen of the stent are compatible with granulation tissue.

stenosis, and local recurrence of malignancy (Figure 2.16). When compared with bronchoscopy, MDCT with 2D multiplanar and 3D reconstruction techniques has been shown to be 88% to 100% sensitive and 100% specific in identifying stent complications. Indeed, MDCT can serve as a noninvasive, highly accurate method for stent surveillance.

SUMMARY

MDCT imaging with 2D multiplanar reformation and 3D reconstruction techniques allows for rapid, noninvasive, and accurate assessment of the tracheobronchial tree. A variety of pathologic processes involving the airways – including airway stenoses, central airway neoplasms, and congenital airway disorders – can be clearly illustrated in a visually accessible manner to the bronchoscopist, thereby providing key information needed for preprocedural planning. The use of dynamic expiratory imaging in conjunction with standard end-inspiratory MDCT imaging is a sensitive technique for the diagnosis of tracheobronchomalacia. MDCT plays an important complementary role to bronchoscopy by

providing critical preprocedural and postprocedural information. MDCT can enhance guidance of bronchoscopic procedures, including sampling of lesions invisible on conventional bronchoscopy. Finally, MDCT is emerging as a primary, noninvasive method for the surveillance of the airways after bronchoscopic interventions, particularly after endoluminal stent placement.

SUGGESTED READINGS

Baroni RH, Feller-Kopman D, Nishino M, Hatabu H, Loring SH, Ernst A, Boiselle PM. Tracheobronchomalacia: comparison between end-expiratory and dynamic expiratory CT for evaluation of central airway collapse. *Radiology*. 2005;235:635–641.

Boiselle PM, Feller-Kopman D, Ashiku S, Weeks D, Ernst A. Tracheobronchomalacia: evolving role of dynamic multislice helical CT. *Radiol Clin North Am*. 2003;41:627–636.

Boiselle PM, Lee KS, Ernst A. Multidetector CT of the central airways. *J Thorac Imaging*. 2005;20:186–195.

Gilkeson RC, Ciancibello LM, Hejal RB, Montenegro HD, Lange P. Tracheobronchomalacia: dynamic airway evaluation with multidetector CT. *AJR Am J Roentgenol*. 2001;176:205–210.

Heyer CM, Nuesslein TG, Jung D, Peters SA, Lemburg SP, Rieger CH, Nicolas V. Tracheobronchial anomalies and stenoses: detection with low-dose multidetector CT with virtual tracheobronchoscopy–comparison with flexible tracheobronchoscopy. *Radiology*. 2007;242:542–549.

Hoppe H, Dinkel HP, Walder B, von Allmen G, Gugger M, Vock P. Grading airway stenosis down to the segmental level using virtual bronchoscopy. *Chest*. 2004;125:704–711.

Lee KS, Lunn W, Feller-Kopman D, Ernst A, Hatabu H, Boiselle PM. Multislice CT evaluation of airway stents. *J Thorac Imaging*. 2005;20:81–88.

Lee KS, Sun MR, Ernst A, Feller-Kopman D, Majid A, Boiselle PM. Comparison of dynamic expiratory CT with bronchoscopy for diagnosing airway malacia: a pilot evaluation. *Chest*. 2007;131:758–764.

McCarthy MJ, Rosado-de-Christenson ML. Tumors of the trachea. *J Thorac Imaging*. 1995;10:180–198.

Quint LE, Whyte RI, Kazerooni EA, Martinez FJ, Cascade PN, Lynch JP 3rd, Orringer MB, Brunsting LA 3rd, Deeb GM. Stenosis of the central airways: evaluation by using helical CT with multiplanar reconstructions. *Radiology*. 1995;194:871–877.

Remy-Jardin M, Remy J, Artaud D, Fribourg M, Duhamel A. Volume rendering of the tracheobronchial tree: clinical evaluation of bronchographic images. *Radiology*. 1998;208:761–770.

Siegel MJ. Multiplanar and three-dimensional multidetector row CT of thoracic vessels and airways in the pediatric population. *Radiology*. 2003;229:641–650.

3

THE LARYNX

Daniel C. Chelius, Jr., and William W. Lunn

"The human voice is the organ of the soul." – Henry Wadsworth Longfellow

INTRODUCTION

The larynx is a complex constricting and dilating gateway to the trachea. The three primary functions of the larynx are (1) protection of the airway, (2) respiration, and (3) phonation. Laryngeal closure also allows the patient to build up intrathoracic pressure (the Valsalva maneuver) prior to coughing. It is essential for physicians performing diagnostic or treatment procedures in or through the upper aerodigestive tract to be familiar with the larynx. The purpose of this chapter is twofold: (1) to discuss laryngeal anatomy and function, and (2) to suggest an approach to laryngeal examination.

ANATOMY

Although it sits on top of the trachea, the larynx is suspended from the sternum, clavicles, skull base, mandible, and anterior vertebral column by a group of extrinsic muscles. Its skeleton is a series of pieces of cartilage held together by ligaments, elastic membranes, and the intrinsic laryngeal muscles.

Cartilages

The cricoid cartilage forms the base of the larynx. Although the larynx is a tubular structure, the cricoid is the only complete cartilaginous ring in the laryngeal skeleton. Thus, injury to the larynx in the region of the cricoid ring from trauma, tumor, or iatrogenic causes may quickly lead to laryngeal collapse and airway obstruction. The cricoid has a signet ring shape and is much taller posteriorly (20–30 mm) than anteriorly (5–7 mm). Whereas the anterior cricoid is palpable below the thyroid cartilage during neck examination, the posterior cricoid rises past the inferior level of the thyroid cartilage (Figure 3.1).

Posteriorly, the cricoid supports the arytenoids (paired, lightweight pyramid-shaped cartilages that are the mobile posterior attachment point for the vocal cords) (Figure 3.2). The cricoarytenoid articulation is a synovial joint that allows the arytenoids to move sideways as well as to slide downward toward the midline. In combination, these movements create the vocal cord abduction (outward movement away from midline) and adduction (inward movement toward midline) essential for proper laryngeal function. Like any other synovial joint, the cricoarytenoid joint is subject to a wide spectrum of pathology including arthritis (infectious or inflammatory), ankylosis (fixation), and dislocation, which can impede vocal cord mobility. The corniculate cartilages sit atop the arytenoids and project posteromedially. During vocal cord adduction, they approach each other in the midline and exert laterally directed elastic recoil on the posterior vocal cords. The cuneiform cartilages are suspended in the aryepiglottic fold and are often

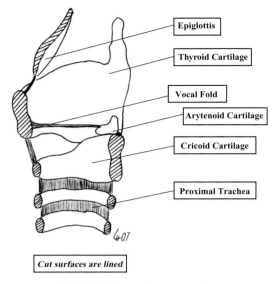

Epiglottis

Thyroid Cartilage

Vocal Fold

Arytenoid Cartilage

Cricoid Cartilage

Proximal Trachea

Cut surfaces are lined

FIGURE 3.1. Larynx in cross section.

visible as raised white masses during endoscopy, sometimes mistaken for malignancy or a submucosal cyst.

The thyroid cartilage is the largest and most prominent laryngeal cartilage. It is shaped like a shield and appropriately named (*thyrus* = shield, Greek) as it protects the internal anatomy of the larynx. The thyroid cartilage has paired superior and inferior horns, or cornua. The superior cornua have ligamentous attachments to the hyoid above, an important part of the laryngeal suspension. The inferior cornua articulate with the lateral cricoid cartilage. This cricothyroid joint is also a synovial joint that allows anteroposterior rocking of the thyroid cartilage on the cricoid;

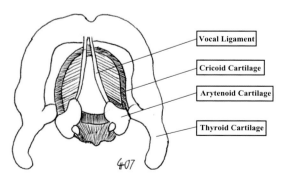

Vocal Ligament

Cricoid Cartilage

Arytenoid Cartilage

Thyroid Cartilage

FIGURE 3.2. Larynx viewed from above.

therefore, it is also susceptible to the pathologies mentioned above.

The epiglottis contains the leaf-shaped epiglottic cartilage that is suspended anteriorly from the hyoid and inferiorly from the thyroid by a series of ligaments. As the larynx tips anterosuperiorly during swallowing, the epiglottic base is pushed against the tongue base, causing the epiglottis to fold over the laryngeal inlet. Although the hyoid is not typically considered part of the larynx, it is intimately associated with the superior cartilages and is important in the laryngeal suspension. The hyoid, thyroid, cricoid, and arytenoids are composed of hyaline cartilage and progressively ossify. The hyoid is completely ossified by age 2; the thyroid begins to ossify in the early 20s, and the cricoid and arytenoids follow shortly thereafter.

Membranes

There are two important submucosal elastic membranes in the larynx: the quadrangular membrane superiorly and the conus elasticus inferiorly. The quadrangular membrane joins the lateral epiglottis, the arytenoids, and the corniculate cartilages. The inferior border joins the vestibular ligament above the vocal fold to form the "false vocal cord," and the superior border and its membranous covering form the aryepiglottic fold. The conus elasticus joins the superior border of the cricoid to the thyroid and arytenoid cartilages. The superior edge of the conus elasticus runs between the midline posterior thyroid cartilage (anterior commissure) and the vocal process of the arytenoids. This free edge is the vocal ligament, the elastic component of the true vocal cord.

Muscles

The intrinsic muscles of the larynx cause the configuration changes in the laryngeal cartilages that open or close and loosen or tighten the vocal cords. The paired thyroarytenoid, lateral cricoarytenoid, and unpaired interarytenoid muscles adduct the vocal cords, whereas the paired posterior cricoarytenoid muscles are the

only abductors. The paired cricothyroid muscles tip the thyroid cartilage anteriorly on the cricoid, tightening the vocal cords further.

The extrinsic muscles of the larynx suspend it in the soft tissues of the neck. The laryngeal elevators raise and anteriorly displace the larynx during swallowing to prevent aspiration. These elevators include the stylohyoid, digastric, and stylopharyngeus from the skull base and the geniohyoid and mylohyoid from the mandible. The elevating forces exerted on the hyoid are transmitted to the larynx by the thyrohyoid muscle and ligaments. The laryngeal depressors displace the larynx downward during inspiration and include the remaining strap muscles – omohyoid, sternohyoid, and sternothyroid. The esophageal constrictors and cricopharyngeus insert on the posterior larynx and are critical to the swallowing reflex.

MUCOSA

The larynx is lined by two different types of mucosa. The free edges of the true vocal cords, upper edges of the aryepiglottic folds, and superior epiglottis are covered in stratified squamous epithelium whereas the remainder of the larynx is covered in pseudostratified ciliated columnar respiratory epithelium. The mucosa is a continuous sheet as it wraps over the top of the epiglottis and reflects onto the tongue base, forming the vallecula. A layer of loose connective tissue is immediately deep to the mucosa in the bulk of the larynx. However, this layer of connective tissue is absent on the laryngeal (posterior) surface of the epiglottis, which accounts for the marked anterior epiglottic swelling that can be seen in epiglottitis or supraglottitis.

The submucosal layers of the vocal cord are completely distinct from the remainder of the larynx and deserve special attention. The vocal cord consists of three main layers: the stratified squamous cover, the trilamellar lamina propria, and the vocalis muscle. The superficial layer of the lamina propria is very loose connective tissue

that has the consistency of a soft gelatin. This is the primary layer in which vibration during phonation occurs and is also the layer most likely to become filled with edematous fluid because of its loose configuration. The intermediate and deep layers of the lamina propria consist of elastic and collagen fibers, respectively. These layers form the vocal ligament and are the termination of the conus elasticus.

INNERVATION

The superior and inferior laryngeal nerves arise from the vagus nerve to innervate the intrinsic muscles and mucosa of the larynx. The superior nerve branches off at the nodose ganglion, passes deep to the carotid artery, runs laterally to the larynx in the submucosa of the piriform sinus, and then divides into internal and external branches. The internal branch pierces the thyrohyoid membrane with the superior laryngeal artery to give sensory and secretory innervation to the laryngeal mucosa above the true vocal cords. The external branch runs laterally to the thyroid cartilage to innervate the cricothyroid muscle. The inferior laryngeal nerve is the termination of the recurrent laryngeal nerve. The recurrent laryngeal nerve branches off the vagus in the chest and wraps around the subclavian artery on the right and the aortic arch on the left before ascending to the tracheoesophageal groove. The inferior nerve pierces the cricothyroid membrane and provides motor innervation to all of the intrinsic muscles except the cricothyroid. The recurrent laryngeal nerve is not well organized internally, so when the nerve is divided, reanastomosis does not typically restore normal motor function.

ENDOSCOPIC LANDMARKS

From a superior vantage point during endoscopic examination of the larynx, there are a number of important landmarks to consider. Starting

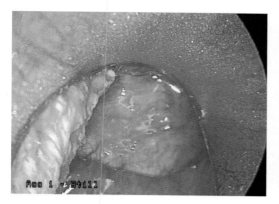

FIGURE 3.3. Tongue base, epiglottis, and vallecula.

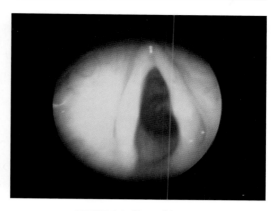

FIGURE 3.4. Normal larynx.

anteriorly, one can see the tongue base, vallecula, and epiglottis in most patients (Figure 3.3). To fully visualize these structures, it may be necessary for the patient to slightly protrude the tongue if he or she suffers from "pharyngeal crowding" or obesity. Moving posterior and inferior, one can see the aryepiglottic folds leading down to the arytenoids with bumps in the mucosa representing the underlying cuneiform and corniculate cartilages. The laryngeal surface of the epiglottis leads down to the anterior commissure at the level of the true vocal cords (Figure 3.4). However, above the true vocal cords is the vestibule, superiorly bound by the false vocal cords (Figure 3.5). The true vocal cords can be divided into the more anterior portion, which is primarily responsible for the vibration leading to

phonation, and the posterior portion. The posterior intercartilaginous area is the site of articulation of the vocal cord with the vocal process of the arytenoid cartilage. The postcricoid space lies behind the larynx, and the piriform sinuses lie laterally. The piriform sinuses are pyramid-shaped with the bases superior at the level of the laryngeal inlet and the apices at the inlet of the esophagus. The piriform apices are not always visible during flexible endoscopic examination. The examiner may ask the patient to puff the cheeks out to better visualize the piriform sinuses during endoscopy. The subglottic larynx is the area below the true cords and is vulnerable to injury, as discussed above.

ENDOSCOPIC EXAMINATION

It is essential for the novice and the expert alike to develop a consistent routine for laryngeal examination to minimize missed findings. A standard vocabulary for describing laryngeal findings will facilitate accurate and efficient communication between specialists. We have found it useful to systematically move through anatomic landmarks while considering a specific set of examination parameters (Table 3.1). The mnemonic ACCMME outlines a helpful examination system.

The first and most critical aspect of laryngeal examination is ensuring a widely patent **airway**.

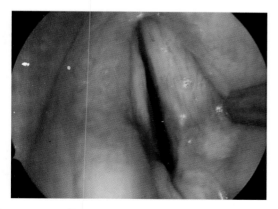

FIGURE 3.5. True and false cords, with a probe in the vestibule.

Table 3.1. *Systematic laryngeal examination*

Anatomic landmarks	Exam parameters (ACCMME)
Tongue base	Airway
Vallecula	Contour
Epiglottis	Color
Aryepiglottic fold	Mucosa
Posterior glottis	Mobility
False vocal cords	Edema
Vestibule	
True vocal cords	
Anterior commissure	
Subglottis	
Piriform sinuses	
Posterior and lateral pharyngeal walls	

Many decisions about subsequent management hinge on the examiner's description of the airway stability. The airway may be obstructed at the larynx from varied etiologies. Each laryngeal examination should include a simple subjective characterization of the airway as widely patent, patent, narrowed, marginal, or critical.

The laryngeal mucosa is typically pink with the exception of the true vocal cords, which should be pearly white. In either of these locations, the **color** should be homogenous. Variability in color may be an early sign of pathology. For example, erythema typically indicates hypervascularity or inflammation that may be a sign of upper respiratory infection, post-tussive laryngitis, early cancer, or acid reflux. In contrast, chronic acid reflux causes a gray discoloration and heaping up of the interarytenoid mucosa known as pachydermia. The true vocal cords may assume a dusky gray color in smokers. Whitish discoloration, also known as leukoplakia, is an early sign of neoplasia. Submucosal vascular lesions may give the mucosa a purple or bluish hue. Overall laryngeal color and the specific location of color abnormalities should be recorded.

Detecting alterations in the **contour** or position of laryngeal structures requires extensive experience with the normal laryngeal examination. Effacement of normal pharyngeal or laryngeal spaces such as the vallecula, piriform sinuses, and vestibule may indicate a submucosal mass, abscess, hematoma, or infiltrative process. More subtle contour changes like asymmetric twisting or tilting of structures may also indicate an infiltrative process. Abnormally sized or absent laryngeal landmarks can also be pathologic. Vallecular effacement may be a surrogate marker for an enlarged tongue base, a contributing factor in obstructive sleep apnea. Neurologic lesions can also result in subtle contour changes. Damage to the external branch of the superior laryngeal nerve causes the larynx to rotate away from the side with the lesion whereas damage to the inferior laryngeal nerve can result in a malpositioned vocal cord. Contour irregularities can be difficult to describe. The description can include position relative to nearby normal landmarks or to the normal larynx as a reference.

The laryngeal **mucosa** is susceptible to the same diseases as any other similar epithelium including carcinoma, bacterial/fungal/viral infections, and inflammatory or autoimmune ulcerations. Because the vocal cords are repeatedly forced together for phonation, coughing, and airway protection, the vocal cord mucosa is prone to trauma-related conditions such as granulomas and contact ulcerations. This is especially true when a patient inappropriately strains the vocal cords through vocal abuse. Traumatic hemorrhage into the vocal cord can occur with such prolonged abuse or with acute severe trauma from yelling or forceful singing. Such a hemorrhage can eventually transform into a vocal cord nodule. Finally, direct trauma to the vocal cords from extrinsic forces such as traumatic or prolonged intubation can result in similar contact-related pathologies. Table 3.2 lists some common mucosal abnormalities with clues to differential diagnosis. Figures 3.6–3.10 provide examples of some of the lesions described in Table 3.2.

All critical laryngeal functions rely on normal laryngeal **mobility**. Examining laryngeal mobility requires more than simply detecting

Table 3.2. *Common laryngeal mucosal abnormalities*

Lesion	Location	Description
Retention cyst	Vallecula, vestibule, undersurface of vocal cord	Unilateral, smooth, filled with clear or straw-colored fluid
Epidermoid cyst	Medial edge of vocal cord	Unilateral, submucosal, smooth, white
Vocal cord nodule	Junction of anterior and middle thirds of cords	Paired; Initially: smooth, soft, red; Mature: hard, white, fibrotic
Vocal cord polyps	Medial edge of vocal cord	Unilateral, pedunculated, fusiform, or diffuse
Contact ulcer	Posterior vocal process of arytenoid	Bilateral, red, ulcerated
Intubation granuloma	Posterior vocal process of arytenoid	Unilateral, red, large, and pedunculated
Papilloma	Vocal cords or vestibule	Heaped up, warty appearance, pink or red, multifocal
Hemangioma	Variable	Purple or blue, submucosal
Squamous cell carcinoma	Variable	Initially: flat whitish plaque with irregular borders; Mature: large, irregular, white or red, ulcerated

vocal cord paralysis. It involves assessing the quality of vocal cord movement and picking up subtle clues about underlying pathology not necessarily visible through the scope. The voice is a sensitive indicator of appropriate vocal fold movement, so this part of the examination begins when first encountering a patient. Many examiners report any abnormal voice as "hoarse." There are many characteristics of an abnormal voice that are more informative than such a catch-all phrase. A voice may be high or low, soft or loud, weak or powerful, breathy or clear, sharp or dull, sonorous or thin, resonant or falsetto, periodic or raw and harsh, relaxed or tense and strained. Various pathologies have typical vocal alterations that essentially fall within

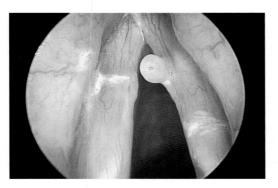

FIGURE 3.6. TVC (true vocal chord) polyp: a smooth, pink, pedunculated lesion of the anterior right vocal cord.

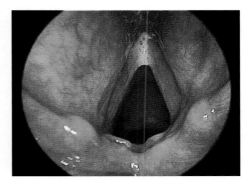

FIGURE 3.7. TVC reflux: laryngeal edema with heaped up mucosa and ulceration over the arytenoids and interarytenoid space.

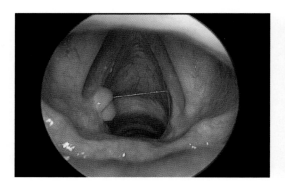

FIGURE 3.8. TVC granuloma: smooth white lesion over the left vocal process.

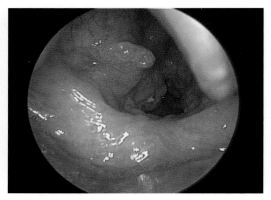

FIGURE 3.9. TVC papillomas: heaped up, smooth, warty lesions disturbing the normal vocal cord contours; involves the supraglottis, glottis, and subglottis.

this set of descriptors. In addition to laryngeal mobility, inadequate breath support from diseased lower airways can also alter the voice and should be considered as well.

The term stridor is used to describe loud upper airway sounds that are generated by turbulent airflow. The examiner should note if stridor, when present, occurs during inspiration, expiration, or both. Although stridor often results from pathology in the larynx, it can also be produced by disease in the upper trachea.

The majority of laryngeal mobility disorders can be diagnosed from history and laryngoscopy with a flexible scope. To assess vocal cord movement, the glottis is examined while the patient phonates. Sustained long vowel sounds at various pitches are best for assessing gross vocal cord movement, whereas short phrases ("every," "each," "Harry likes hamburgers") are best for assessing coordination. When an abnormality in vocal cord movement is detected, asking the patient to count as high as possible on one breath gives a baseline idea of how much the abnormality affects breath control.

The vocal cords rest in the abducted position approximately 25° from the midline and move symmetrically toward the midline during phonation. A completely immobile vocal cord may be paralyzed by denervation, fixed by some infiltrative process, or fixed due to cricoarytenoid joint disease. The paralyzed cord will typically rest in the midline with a bowed appearance whereas the fixed cord may be in any position, bowed or taut, depending on the underlying pathology. In either case, the contralateral vocal fold may cross the midline, making contact with the immobile cord and preserving better laryngeal function than would be expected. Additionally, the false vocal folds may be voluntarily or involuntarily used to phonate, especially in the case of a unilateral vocal cord paralysis. This is called plica ventricularis, and it can make assessment of the vocal cord mobility much more difficult. Frequently, laryngeal examination reveals a problem with vocal cord movement less severe than outright immobility. This can be described as weakness or paresis.

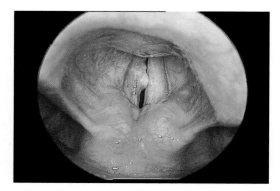

FIGURE 3.10. TVC cancer: irregular white lesion of the left vocal cord.

Finally, the larynx should be carefully examined for **edema**, which may be mild in the case of acid reflux or possibly life threatening in the cases of supraglottitis or angioedema. Vocal cord edema (Reinke's edema) is most frequently seen in women with hypothyroidism or in smokers. However, this is usually not a life-threatening situation and can be managed medically. Careful note should be made of the exact laryngeal structures that are edematous so that improvement or worsening can be documented with serial examinations.

CONCLUSION

The larynx is a complex and elegant organ; it is not something to "get past in order to do the bronchoscopy." Many decisions about airway management hinge on the status of the larynx. A proper understanding of laryngeal anatomy and function is necessary for one to become an expert bronchoscopist.

ACKNOWLEDGMENTS

We are grateful to Luise Holzhauser, our medical student, for drawing the pictures of the laryngeal anatomy that appear in this text. We are also grateful to Dr. Richard Stasney, who kindly provided some of the photographs of laryngeal pathology.

SUGGESTED READINGS

Hirano M, Kiminori S. *Histological Color Atlas of the Human Larynx.* San Francisco: Singular Publishing Group, Inc.; 1993.

Hurley R. *The Larynx: A Multidisciplinary Approach, 2nd ed.* St. Louis: Mosby; 1996.

Lehmann W, Pidoux JM, Widmann JJ. *Larynx: Microlaryngoscopy and Histopathology.* Cadempino, Switzerland: Inpharzam SA; 1981.

Sasaki CT, Kim TH. Anatomy and physiology of the larynx. In: *Ballenger's Otorhinolaryngology Head and Neck Surgery, 16th ed.* Ontario: BC Decker Inc.; 2003:1090–1109.

Yanagisawa E. *Color Atlas of Diagnostic Endoscopy in Otorhinolaryngology.* New York: Igaku-Shoin Medical Publishers; 1997.

4

AIRWAY ANATOMY FOR THE BRONCHOSCOPIST

Rani Kumaran, Arthur Sung, and Armin Ernst

INTRODUCTION

Bronchoscopy is a diagnostic and therapeutic procedure that permits direct visualization of normal and pathological alterations of the upper and lower airways. Expert knowledge of airway anatomy is a prerequisite for successful performance of the procedure. The major advantages of the flexible bronchoscope (FB) include the ability to insert it nasally, orally, or through a tracheostomy stoma to visualize apical segments of upper lobes as well as segmental and subsegmental bronchi in all lobes. This chapter focuses on identification of normal anatomy, landmarks, and pathologies seen during bronchoscopy of upper airways (from nares to glottis) and lower airways (trachea and conducting bronchi).

Bronchoscopists commonly refer to airway anatomy according to the Jackson–Huber classification with segmental airway anatomy named according to spatial orientation (i.e., anterior/posterior, superior/inferior, and medial/lateral) (Figure 4.1) Table 4.1 lists the nomenclature accordingly. Many thoracic surgeons prefer to use the Boyden surgical classification, which assigns numbers to the segmental airways (Table 4.1). It is advised that beginning bronchoscopists learn the Jackson–Huber classification first, emphasizing accurate and consistent usage.

The FB is introduced by the bronchoscopist standing either behind the head of the supine patient or facing the patient. The anatomic orientation of airways varies depending on the operator's position. For the purpose of consistency in this chapter, the anatomical orientation is presented with the operator standing behind the supine patient.

UPPER AIRWAY

Nasopharynx

The upper airway examination begins with a quick assessment of nasal and oral cavities. When the FB is introduced through the nose, the inferior turbinate is seen laterally and the nasal septum is seen medially. The bronchoscope is then directed posteriorly into the pharynx. When viewing the nasal cavity, the bronchoscopist should assess for septal deviation, hypertrophy of turbinates, presence of polyps, and integrity of mucosa. Serosanguineous nasal drainage with severe crusting may be suggestive of Wegener's granulomatosis. Isolated, large septal perforation with inflamed and crusty edges is highly suggestive of nasal substance abuse. Diffuse nasal crusting or a vasomotor-like appearance to the nasal mucosa can typify sarcoidosis. In appropriate clinical settings, nasal polyps may suggest cause for postnasal drip and reactive airway

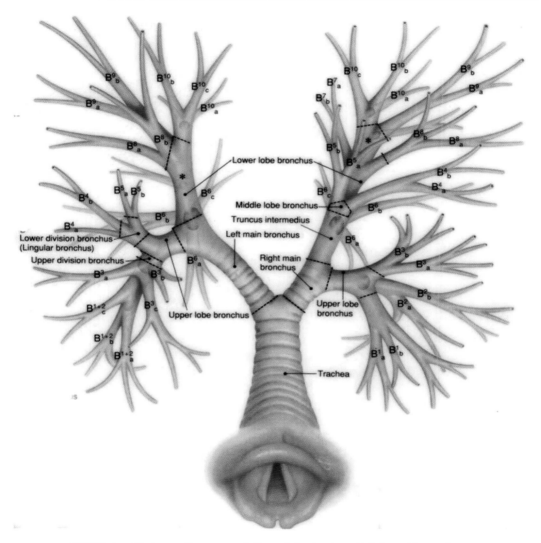

Lower lobe bronchus

Middle lobe bronchus
Truncus intermedius
Left main bronchus

Lower division bronchus
(Lingular bronchus)

Upper division bronchus

Right main
bronchus

Upper lobe
bronchus

Upper lobe bronchus

Trachea

FIGURE 4.1. Diagrammatic representation of tracheobronchial tree. The authors acknowledge Olympus Company for providing Figure 4.1.

diseases, such as atopic asthma or vasculitides (e.g., Churg–Strauss syndrome). Nasal tuberculosis may show a red, nodular thickening, with or without ulceration. A rapidly progressive black, necrotic mass of tissue filling the nasal cavity, eroding the nasal septum, and extending through the hard palate characterizes mucormycosis.

Oropharynx and Hypopharynx

When the FB is introduced orally, it passes through the oropharynx and larynx and into the trachea. Beyond the base of the tongue, the bronchoscope is passed through the curvature of the oropharynx, which is bordered superiorly by the soft palate and extends to the tip of the epiglottis. The FB is then directed posterior to the tip of the epiglottis. The three major structures in the hypopharynx are the pyriform recess, the postcricoid region, and the posterior pharyngeal wall (Figure 4.2). Tongue size, tooth integrity, and temporomandibular joint mobility are important factors affecting the ease

Table 4.1. *Boyden surgical classification / Jackson–Huber classification*

Right bronchial tree		Left bronchial tree	
RUL		LUL	
B1	Apical	Upper division	
B2	Posterior	B1/2	Apicoposterior
B3	Anterior	B3	Anterior
RML		Lingular	
B4	Lateral	B4	Superior
B5	Medial	B5	Inferior
RLL		LLL	
B6	Superior	B6	Superior
B7	Medial basal	B7/8	Anteromedial
B8	Anterior basal	B9	Lateral basal
B9	Lateral basal	B10	Posterior basal
B10	Posterior		

Note: RUL, right upper lobe; LUL, left upper lobe; RML, right middle lobe; RLL, right lower lobe; LLL, left lower lobe.

of introduction into the oropharynx. The space between the base of the tongue and the anterior surface of the epiglottis on either side constitutes the vallecula. The valleculae are separated by the median glossoepiglottic fold and bordered laterally on either side by the lateral glossoepiglottic folds. Valleculae are often locations for foreign body entrapment and upper airway obstruction.

Larynx

The bronchoscopist should assess the vocal cords for normal abduction on inspiration and adduction during phonation. Dysfunction of vocal cords can be either functional or organic, as seen in persistent gastroesophageal acid reflux, and can cause significant airway compromise. Paradoxical vocal cord motion is an inappropriate adduction of the true vocal cords throughout the respiratory cycle with the obliteration of glottic aperture except for a posterior diamond-shaped opening.

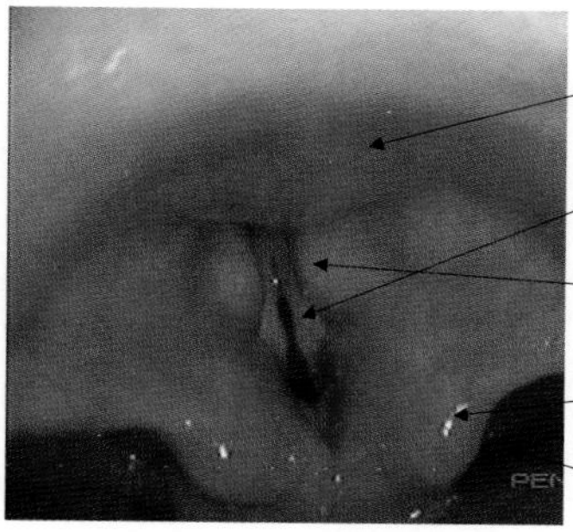

The glossopharyngeal nerve and the vagus nerve supply the motor and sensory pathways for the larynx. The superior laryngeal branch of the vagus nerve (SLN) provides sensory innervation to the glottis, the arytenoids, and the vocal cords. Stimulation of pathways of the SLN, including manipulation of pyriform recess, may result in protective closure of the glottis. Therefore, it is paramount that appropriate topical anesthesia to theses structures be applied prior to proceeding with bronchoscopy.

LOWER AIRWAY

- Base of the epiglottis
- True vocal cords
- Vestibular fold
- Arytenoids
- Pyriform sinus

FIGURE 4.2 Laryngeal anatomy.

Trachea

The lower airway (trachea to conductive bronchi) begins at the cricoid cartilage (at about the level of the sixth cervical vertebra, C6). The adult trachea ranges from 16 to 20 mm in internal diameter

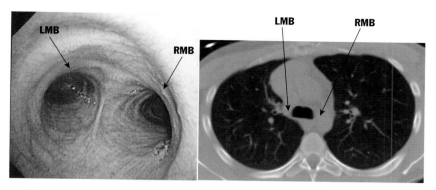

FIGURE 4.3. Carina with right and left main bronchus. (RMB, right main bronchus; LMB, left main bronchus)

and has 18–22 cartilage rings. The trachea tapers slightly and aims posteriorly as it divides at the carina, at the level of fifth thoracic spine to the left and right main stem bronchi. The horseshoe-shaped tracheal cartilage shapes the anterior part of the trachea, whereas the posterior part of the trachea consists of smooth muscles that joins the ends of the tracheal cartilage (Figure 4.3).

Starting at the upper trachea, mucosal integrity should be examined, even when there are no gross endobronchial lesions. The presence of extrinsic tracheal deviation and compression due to paratracheal masses should be noted. Both the anterior cartilaginous and posterior membranous portions of the trachea are sometimes sites for dynamic airway compromise caused by tracheomalacia or excessive dynamic airway collapse. The distal trachea and main carina are important sites for examination because malignant diseases often metastasize to the surrounding mediastinal lymph nodes.

If a lesion is identified, both sides of the lungs should be examined completely before biopsies are taken. The importance of complete surveillance is that unexpected satellite airway pathologies can occur in up to 10% of primary bronchogenic carcinomas. After main pathology is visualized or diagnostic procedures are started, the bronchoscopist can become too distracted to return to a thorough and careful examination of the remainder of the airways. Furthermore, when the site of primary pathology is sampled,

bleeding can degrade the quality of the FB image, and coughing and oxygen desaturation will limit the time to complete the procedure. There is also a danger that samples retrieved from a secondary site that appear abnormal and are found to contain malignant cells can actually represent contamination from cells dislodged during earlier examination of a primary malignant site. Such false-positive results may have a devastating effect of overstaging a potentially curable peripheral lesion.

Main Carina

The main carina is a keel-shaped structure oriented anteroposteriorly. On flexible bronchoscopy and chest computed tomography (CT), as seen in Figure 4.3, the main carina is identified as a thin septum separating the right and left main bronchi. It is usually sharp in adults, and its dimensions vary during inhalation and exhalation. The angle of the left main carina is usually 10°–15° higher than the right main carina on CT.

Right Bronchial Tree

The right main bronchus is approximately 1.5 cm in length and has an internal diameter of 10–12 mm. The first branch, the right upper lobe (RUL) bronchus, arises just below the carina, and courses laterally for a distance of 1–2 cm before branching into apical, anterior, and posterior segments as seen in Figure 4.4 in flexible bronchoscopy and chest CT. On a CT scan, the

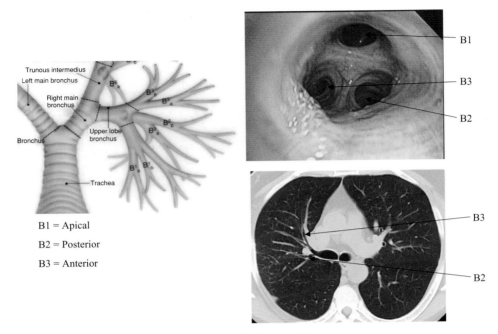

B1 = Apical

B2 = Posterior

B3 = Anterior

FIGURE 4.4. Right upper lobe.

branching point of the RUL bronchus can be identified as a faint curvilinear density marginating the lateral wall of the right main bronchus. The horizontal course of the RUL bronchus with origins of anterior and posterior segments gives the inverted whale tail appearance. These branching points are frequent sites of bronchial disease, including carcinoma. On CT imaging, at the level of distal trachea, the apical segment appears as a circular lucency in proximity to pulmonary vessels. Both anterior and posterior (and their subsegments) can be easily seen.

Beyond the RUL bronchus, the right main bronchus becomes the bronchus intermedius, extends approximately 2–2.5 cm, and divides into right middle lobe and lower lobe bronchi as seen in Figure 4.5 in flexible bronchoscopy and chest CT. In chest CT, the bronchus intermedius is characteristically seen on several adjacent sections. It has an oblique shape and courses directly posterior to the right main pulmonary artery and the right interlobar pulmonary artery inferiorly. A cardiac bronchus, a rare congenital anomaly, can be seen arising from the medial wall of the bronchus intermedius before the origin of the superior segmental branch of the right lower lobe.

The right middle lobe bronchus arises from the anterolateral wall of the bronchus intermedius and extends anteriorly and laterally for about 1–2 cm before dividing into medial and lateral segments. The lateral segmental bronchus is visualized over a greater distance, and the medial segment has a more oblique course. Beyond the origin of the superior segment, the right lower lobe divides into anterior, posterior, medial, and lateral segments as seen Figure 4.6 in flexible bronchoscopy and chest CT.

Left Bronchial Tree

The left main bronchus is approximately 4–4.5 cm in length and tends to progress posteriorly, inferiorly, and laterally. It divides into left upper and lower lobe bronchi as seen in Figure 4.7 on flexible bronchoscopy and chest CT. The left main bronchus is much longer than the right and is radiologically seen in three to four contiguous sections below the carina. The

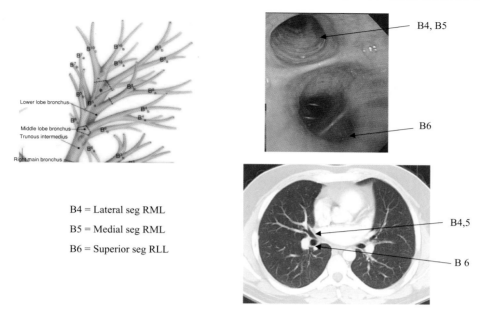

B4 = Lateral seg RML

B5 = Medial seg RML

B6 = Superior seg RLL

FIGURE 4.5. Right middle lobe and right lower lobe.

upper lobe bronchus is 2- to 3-cm long and divides into upper lobe and lingular divisions. The origin of the left upper lobe bronchus forms a sling over which the left main pulmonary artery passes. The upper lobe division divides into apicoposterior and anterior segmental bronchi as seen in Figure 4.8 on flexible bronchoscopy and chest CT. The anterior segmental bronchus is directed anteriorly and accompanied by the anterior segmental artery. As the

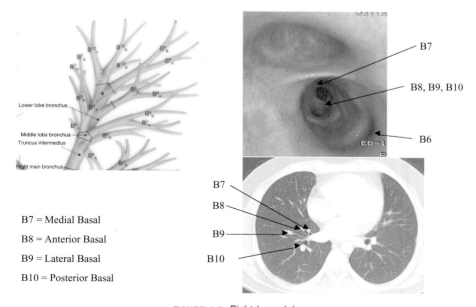

B7 = Medial Basal

B8 = Anterior Basal

B9 = Lateral Basal

B10 = Posterior Basal

FIGURE 4.6. Right lower lobe.

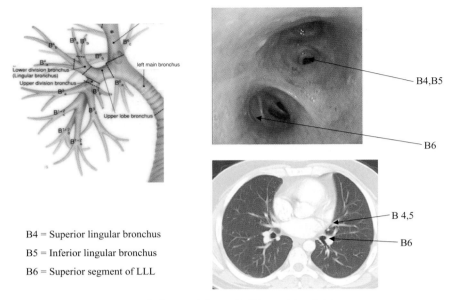

B4 = Superior lingular bronchus

B5 = Inferior lingular bronchus

B6 = Superior segment of LLL

FIGURE 4.7. Left upper lobe and left lower lobe division.

upper lobe bronchus extends superiorly, the lingular branch arises and extends slightly downward in an inferolateral direction. The lingular bronchus is about 2–3 cm in length and divides into superior and inferior segmental bronchi.

The superior segment of the left lower lobe bronchus arises immediately on entering into

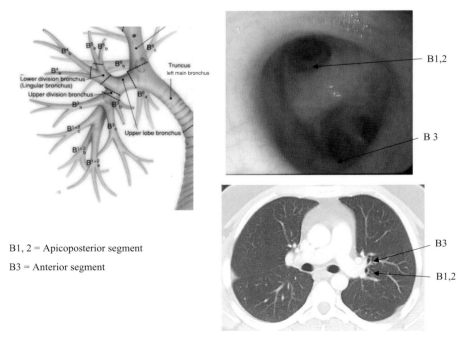

B1, 2 = Apicoposterior segment

B3 = Anterior segment

FIGURE 4.8. Left upper lobe.

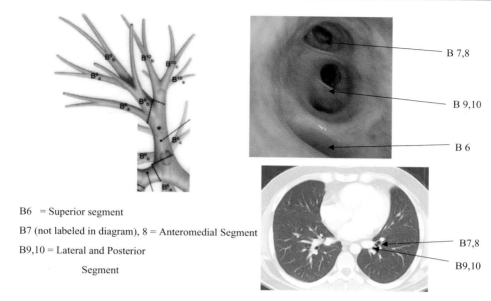

B6 = Superior segment

B7 (not labeled in diagram), 8 = Anteromedial Segment

B9,10 = Lateral and Posterior

       Segment

FIGURE 4.9. Basilar segment of left lower lobe.

the left lower lobe as seen in Figure 4.7 on flexible bronchoscopy and chest CT. Beyond this, the left lower lobe bronchi is approximately 1 cm in length and divides into anteromedial, lateral, and posterior basilar segments as seen in Figure 4.9 on flexible bronchoscopy and chest CT.

CONCLUSION

Solid knowledge of normal and variations in normal tracheobronchial anatomy is the key for successful bronchoscopy. Composite knowledge of adjacent pulmonary vasculature and mediastinal and other structures will aid in performance of specialized diagnostic and therapeutic bronchoscopic procedures.

SUGGESTED READINGS

Boiselle PM. Imaging of the large airways; *Clin Chest Med.* 2008;29(1):181–193.

Letko E. Relapsing polychondritis: a clinical review. *Semin Arthritis Rheum.* 2002;31:384.

Mani SK, Mehta A. Applied anatomy of the airways. In: Wang KP, Mehta AC, Turner JF, eds. *Flexible Bronchoscopy, Part I: Fundamentals of Bronchoscopy, 2nd ed.* Hoboken, NJ: Wiley-Blackwell; 2003;36–38.

Marks SC, Pasha R. *Rhinology and Paranasal Sinuses, Otolaryngology: Head and Neck Surgery. A Clinical and Reference Guide, 2nd ed.* San Diego: Plural Publishing; 2005.

McDonald TJ. Vasculitis and granulomatous disease. In: McCaffrey TV, ed. *Rhinologic Diagnosis and Treatment.* New York: Thieme;1996.

Sung, A, Williams K, Kovitz K. Endotracheal intubation and tracheostomy. In: Fein AM, Kamholz S, Ost D, eds. *Respiratory Emergencies.* London: Hodder Arnold; 2007;41–56.

5

ANESTHESIA FOR BRONCHOSCOPY

John Pawlowski and Stephen D. Pratt

Instrumentation of the airway is among the most noxious procedures physicians perform. Laryngoscopy and tracheal intubation require 1.3–2.8 times more inhalation anesthesia than does surgical incision. Physiologic responses to bronchoscopy include hypertension, tachycardia, increased cardiac output, laryngospasm, bronchospasm, retching, and vomiting. These hemodynamic and respiratory changes may be well tolerated by healthy individuals, but can lead to myocardial ischemia or respiratory compromise in others. To safely and effectively perform bronchoscopy and other airway procedures, pulmonary specialists must be able to adequately anesthetize the upper airway with local anesthetics, and safely administer moderate (conscious) sedation. This chapter will describe the methods used to anesthetize the oropharynx and upper airway, and the safe use of sedative hypnotics to minimize the frequency and severity of these complications.

AIRWAY ANESTHESIA

Neuroanatomy of the Airway

Branches of the Vth, IXth, and Xth cranial nerves provide sensation to the airway. The nasal mucosa is innervated by the sphenopalatine plexus, composed of branches of the maxillary branch of the trigeminal nerve. These fibers lie just below the mucosa along the lateral wall of the nares, posterior to the middle turbinate. Sensation to the anterior 2/3 of the tongue is provided by fibers of the mandibular branch of cranial nerve V. The posterior 1/3 of the tongue and the pharyngeal mucosa to the vocal cords are innervated by the glossopharyngeal nerve through the pharyngeal plexus. The superior laryngeal and recurrent laryngeal branches of the vagus innervate the vocal cords, trachea, and bronchi.

Local Anesthetic Techniques

Many of the nerves of the airway can be directly anesthetized by injection or topical application of local anesthetics. Direct injection of the sphenopalatine plexus nerves can be accomplished by injecting 2–3 mL of local anesthetic below the nasal mucosa just posterior to the middle turbinate. However, this technique is impractical and runs the risk of intravascular injection. It also can lead to blood in the airway, obscuring fiber-optic visualization. More commonly, local anesthesia-soaked pledgets or cotton packing is pressed against the mucosa, anesthetizing the underlying nerves. A cotton swab is introduced into the nares and advanced along the turbinate all the way to the posterior wall of the nasal passage. A second swab is then advanced angled slightly more cephalad to the first along the middle turbinate. This swab is more likely to block the sphenopalatine plexus. These pledgets should be kept in place for 2–3 minutes to allow sub-mucosal penetration of the local anesthetic. A 4% cocaine solution has traditionally been used for this procedure because of its vasoconstrictive properties, but lidocaine works as well.

The glossopharyngeal nerve can be similarly blocked by either injection or topical admin-istration of local anesthetic at the base of the posterior tonsillar pillar (palatopharyngeal fold). After careful aspiration to prevent injection into the nearby carotid artery, approximately 5 mL of local anesthetic are injected into the submu-cosa. A 22-gauge, 9-cm needle is used, and the last 1 cm is bent to facilitate injection behind the pillar. Alternatively, cotton pledgets soaked in local anesthetics can be placed at the base of the posterior tonsillar pillar. Care must be taken not to inject too anteriorly, or the hypoglossal nerve can be blocked and motor function of the tongue impaired.

The internal branch of the superior laryngeal nerve can be blocked where it pierces the thyrohy-oid membrane, halfway between the hyoid bone and the superior border of the thyroid cartilage. With the patient's neck extended, the hyoid bone is moved laterally. The overlying skin is prepped with an alcohol wipe. A 25-gauge, 2.5-cm needle is advanced until it contacts the superior cornu of the hyoid bone, and is then walked off the cornu inferiorly. It is then advanced another 2–3 mm. As the needle passes through the thyrohyoid membrane, a loss of resistance or "pop" is felt. At that point, approximately 3 mL of local anesthe-tic are injected deep and superficial to the mem-brane. Alternatively, the needle can be advanced until air is aspirated and then withdrawn to the submucosal space and the medication injected. The procedure is then repeated on the contralat-eral side. Care must be taken to avoid intravas-cular injection into the carotid artery.

Finally, the trachea can be anesthetized by injection of lidocaine through the cricothyroid membrane. With the patient supine, the skin over the membrane is sanitized with an alco-hol wipe, and a 22- or 20-gauge needle is used to puncture the membrane. Approximately 4 mL of 2% lidocaine is then quickly injected during maximal exhalation. Although this technique is simple and very effective, hemorrhage and even death have been reported because of laceration of small arteries in the cricothyroid membrane.

Although the nerve blocks and injections described above are all effective, they require multiple steps and can be unpleasant for the patient. Therefore, techniques that simply deliver the local anesthetics topically to the mucosa of the airway are more common. Several such tech-niques exist. First, the patient can be asked to gargle and "swish" a 2% viscous lidocaine solu-tion. This technique can effectively anesthetize the tongue, mouth, and posterior pharynx. Alter-natively, a nebulizer can be used to deliver aerosolized local anesthetic from the mouth to the lungs. Approximately 10 mL of 4% lido-caine are administered through a standard neb-ulizer. This technique is well tolerated, effective as the sole technique in 50% of patients, and may be associated with lower plasma levels com-pared with direct endobronchial administration; however, nebulized lidocaine may not decrease the amount of supplemental lidocaine needed by direct, endobronchial injection, and high serum levels have been described with this technique. Various sprays and atomizers can be used to directly spray the posterior pharynx. After the tongue has been sprayed, it can be grasped with gauze and the spray device inserted into the posterior pharynx. The patient is asked to take deep breaths, and local anesthetic is sprayed dur-ing inspiration. Commercially available products can be used to administer benzocaine, or a stan-dard atomizer can be filled with lidocaine for this technique.

Finally, the bronchoscopist can simply use the "spray-as-you-go" method, administering the local anesthetic through the working port of the scope. Lidocaine (4%) is used most frequently above the vocal cords with this method, whereas 2% lidocaine is generally used below the cords. One report found this technique superior to neb-ulized lidocaine. All of the techniques described

Table 5.1. *Local anesthetics*

Drug	Maximum dose	Concerns
Lidocaine	• 4–9 mg/kg (37,40) • 200–400 mg max dose (25,87) • <175 mg/m^2 (20)	• Seizures • Ventricular tachydysrhythmias • Sedation
Benzocaine	1–2 s spray of Cetacaine or Hurricane (9)	• Methemoglobinemia
Cocaine	1 mg/kg (4)	• Hypertension • Tachycardia • Myocardial ischemia and infarction

above for anesthetizing the airway are effective and safe when properly employed. Comparisons between them have not demonstrated that one is clearly superior to another.

Local Anesthetic Drugs and Their Complications

Several local anesthetics have been described for airway anesthesia, including lidocaine, tetracaine, benzocaine, and cocaine (see Table 5.1). Of these, 2% and 4% lidocaine are the most common. Irrespective of the technique used for airway anesthesia, the bronchoscopist must be vigilant in watching for signs and symptoms of local anesthetics toxicity. During a nerve block technique, the intra-arterial injection of even a small amount of local anesthetic into the carotid artery can cause seizures and other central nervous system (CNS) toxicity. Topical techniques can lead to the absorption of large quantities of the local anesthetic and to systemic toxicity. The signs and symptoms of local anesthetic toxicity are described in Table 5.2. When doses of

300–400 mg of lidocaine are used, serum lidocaine levels are generally well below toxic levels. The serum concentration is directly related to the dose of local anesthetic administered, and symptoms generally occur when the serum level is >5 mg/L. However, clinicians frequently administer more than the recommended doses without apparent complications, with doses exceeding 600 mg being described. The apparent relative safety of these larger doses is probably due to the fact that 88%–92% of the drug administered by a nebulizer is wasted. Nonetheless, high serum lidocaine levels, seizures, and even death from local anesthetic toxicity have been described.

The use of benzocaine spray or cocaine solution raises other specific concerns. Benzocaine metabolism in the blood can lead to the formation of methemoglobinemia. Although this is a relatively rare complication, severe cyanosis, arterial desaturation to levels below 40%, and death have been reported. Methemoglobin levels above 30% are common. Use of a benzocaine spray (compared with other gel or solution applications) increases the likelihood of methemoglobinemia, and it has been described after only a single spray. Treatment includes supplemental oxygen and intravenous (IV) methylene blue (1 mg/kg). Cocaine is frequently used for topical anesthesia of the nose. Its effects on the cardiovascular system are well known. Myocardial ischemia and infarction have been described after topical cocaine administration to the airway.

The administration of anticholinergic agents, such as atropine or glycopyrrolate, is frequently

Table 5.2. *Signs and symptoms of local anesthetic toxicity*

Early signs and symptoms	Late signs and symptoms
Metallic taste	Somnolence
Tinnitus	Sedation
Anxiety	Seizure
Light-headedness	Ventricular arrhythmia (V. Tach and V. Fib) Cardiovascular collapse

recommended to decrease secretions, improve visibility, and enhance the efficacy of topical local anesthetics. Although this practice is not recommended prior to bronchoscopy, it remains common. Randomized trials have demonstrated that these medications do not improve the quality of airway anesthesia or bronchoscopic view. Higher serum lidocaine concentrations have been reported after the use of atropine. Clinicians should be wary of the potential complications from the tachycardia caused by these medications.

MODERATE SEDATION

Introduction

Adequate local anesthesia allows the clinician to perform flexible, fiber-optic bronchoscopy without the addition of sedatives or anxiolytics, and the concomitant administration of moderate (conscious) sedation during this procedure is controversial. Conflicting data exist as to whether sedation improves patient tolerance of the procedure. In addition, many of the complications associated with bronchoscopy, and up to 1/2 of the life-threatening events can be attributed to the sedation. Others have suggested that sedation should be routine for bronchoscopy. Irrespective of this controversy, a large majority of physicians routinely administer sedation during bronchoscopy. Thus, it is incumbent on the bronchoscopist to understand the regulatory requirements, risks, benefits, medication dosages, monitoring requirements, and impact of patient disease states to safely administer moderate sedation.

Definition and Oversight

Many local, state, and national agencies have published recommendations, guidelines, and standards for the administration of sedation. The clinician must become familiar with these regulations and any local hospital policies regulating the practice of sedation. The American Society of Anesthesiologists (ASA) has published

guidelines for the administration of sedation and analgesia by nonanesthesiologists. These guidelines define a continuum of sedation depth, ranging from minimal sedation (anxiolysis) to general anesthesia, as described below.

- **Anxiolysis:** A drug-induced state during which patients respond normally to verbal commands. Although cognitive function and coordination may be impaired, ventilator and cardiovascular functions are unaffected.
- **Moderate sedation/analgesia (previously called conscious sedation):** A drug-induced depression of consciousness during which patients respond purposefully to verbal commands, either alone or accompanied by light tactile stimulation. No interventions are required to maintain a patent airway, and spontaneous ventilation is adequate. Cardiovascular function is usually maintained (withdrawal from a noxious stimulus is not purposeful movement).
- **Deep sedation:** A drug-induced depression of consciousness during which patients cannot be easily aroused but respond purposefully following repeated painful stimulation. The ability to independently maintain ventilatory function may be impaired. Patients may require assistance in maintaining a patent airway, and spontaneous ventilation may be inadequate. Cardiovascular function is usually maintained (withdrawal from a noxious stimulus is not purposeful movement).
- **General anesthesia:** A drug-induced loss of consciousness during which patients are not awakened, even by painful stimuli.

The ASA guideline outlines recommendations for preprocedure patient evaluation, patient monitoring, equipment availability, training of personnel, drug administration, and the recovery and discharge of patients during moderate or deep sedation. A full review of these guidelines is beyond the scope of this chapter, but the pulmonary physician should be familiar with its contents. In addition, The Joint Commission has adopted many of the recommendations of the ASA guideline and uses the same definitions for moderate and deep sedation. Furthermore, nine Joint Commission standards apply directly to the administration of sedation. All clinicians who administer sedation for interventional pulmonary procedures in the United States must comply with these standards:

- **Moderate or deep sedation is provided by qualified personnel.** This indicates that all personnel who administer sedation must be trained in and have privileges for the safe administration of the sedative medications. In addition, they must be trained to rescue the patient from a deeper than expected level of sedation. Advanced Cardiac Life Support (ACLS) training generally fulfills this requirement.
- **Sedation risks and options are discussed prior to administration.** Clinicians frequently include informed consent for sedation on the form for the procedure.
- **A presedation assessment is performed.** This includes a history and physical examination, evidence that the patient is NPO (*nil per os*, i.e., nothing by mouth) in accordance with guidelines, and specific comorbidities that might impact the safe conduct of the sedation are identified. It also includes a determination that the patient is an appropriate candidate for the procedure and sedation and an immediate preinduction reassessment.
- **Moderate or deep sedation is planned.** Many clinicians create a set of sedation orders that they can complete prior to the procedure.
- **Each patient's physiologic status is monitored during sedation.** See section on monitoring.
- **Each patient's postprocedure status is assessed on admission to and before discharge from the postsedation recovery area.**
- **Patients are discharged from the postsedation recovery area by a licensed, independent practitioner (LIP) or according to criteria approved by the medical staff.** Most institutions create specific, objective criteria

for discharge home or to an inpatient unit for patients who receive sedation. These criteria should include an adult escort home and postsedation instructions (including 24-hour contact information). The clinician must be aware that he or she is still responsible for the safe discharge of the patient, even if the patient has been sent home by a nurse in accordance with hospital criteria.

- **Each patient's physiologic status while undergoing moderate or deep sedation is collected and analyzed.** Many institutions have created a form, much like an anesthesia record, for documenting the conduct of moderate or deep sedation.
- **Outcomes of patients undergoing moderate or deep sedation are collected and analyzed.**

Many other organizations, including the American Association of Respiratory Care, the Association of Operating Room Nurses, the American College of Emergency Physicians, and others, have published guidelines and standards regarding sedation to which the pulmonary physician may be held.

Preprocedure Assessment

The ASA moderate sedation guidelines and The Joint Commission standards require that all patients undergoing moderate or deep sedation have a presedation medical assessment. In addition to a standard history and physical examination, this assessment should include information specific to the safe conduct of moderate sedation:

- Evidence that the patient is NPO in accordance with recommended guidelines
- Assessment of the airway (see below)
- Determination of the ASA Physical Status score (see below)
- Evaluation for abnormalities of any major organ system that could negatively impact the safe conduct of sedation
- Determination that the patient has an adult escort home (for those undergoing an outpatient procedure)

Table 5.3. *ASA physical status*

ASA class	Definition	Examples
Class I	No organic, physiologic, biochemical, or physical disturbances. Process for which the procedure is being performed is localized	Healthy patient
Class II	Mild to moderate systemic disturbance caused either by the condition to be treated or other process	Controlled hypertension, mild asthma, AODM, stable (mild) CAD
Class III	Severe systemic disturbance from whatever cause. Impacts daily function	CAD, COPD, compensated CHF, SLE
Class IV	Life-threatening systemic disturbance	Unstable CAD, end-stage renal failure, severe CHF/COPD, long-standing IDDM with end-organ involvement
Class V	Moribund. Not expected to survive 24 h with or without therapy	Ruptured AAA, gunshot wound, severe sepsis

Note: AODM, adult-onset diabetes mellitus; CAD, coronary artery disease; COPD, chronic obstructive pulmonary disease; CHF, congestive heart failure; SLE, systemic lupus erythematosus; IDDM, insulin-dependent diabetes mellitus; AAA, abdominal aortic aneurysm.

■ History of adverse experience with sedation
■ Consent for sedation (this may be included in the procedural consent)

Assessment of the airway is important because it helps identify those patients in whom endotracheal intubation may be difficult or impossible if they were to become oversedated. The Mallampati classification is one way to identify patients who might be difficult to intubate. To perform this evaluation, ask the patient to open his or her mouth fully and extend the tongue without phonating. The classification is as follows:

■ Class I: The entire tonsillar pillars are visible, as is the posterior pharynx
■ Class II: The top half of the tonsillar pillars can be seen
■ Class III: The tonsillar pillars cannot be seen, but the base of the uvula is visible
■ Class IV: Only the hard palate can be seen

Other physical markers of a potentially difficult intubation include a receding mandible, limited mouth opening (<3.5 cm between upper and lower incisors), pronounced overbite of the maxillary incisors, a decreased thyromental distance, and a history of a difficult or failed intubation. Patients deemed to be at significantly increased risk for difficult intubation may benefit from having an anesthesiologist perform the procedural sedation.

The physician who administers moderate or deep sedation must also understand the impact that comorbid diseases may have on the safe conduct of the sedation. Although fiber-optic bronchoscopy with sedation has been performed on patients with significant comorbidities, including obesity, pregnancy, brain lesions, and coronary disease, having such concurrent medical conditions increases the likelihood of complications from the sedation. A full review of the impact of coexisting disease on sedation is beyond the scope of this chapter, but several points can be made. First, the ASA Physical Status should be determined for each patient receiving moderate or deep sedation (see Table 5.3). Perioperative and anesthesia-related mortality correlates well with increasing ASA class. Many institutions restrict the administration of

Table 5.4. *Risk for complications from sedation*

Comorbidity	Sedation risk
Obesity/sleep apnea	• Central sensitivity to sedatives • Rapid arterial desaturation • Difficulty with mask ventilation or intubation
Hypertension	• Increased rate of hypertension • Exaggerated hypotension from vasodilating effect of medications
Systolic cardiac dysfunction	• Slow circulatory time. Delayed effects of sedatives • Prone to pulmonary edema with IV fluids or hemodynamic consequences of bronchoscopy
Ischemic heart disease	• Myocardial ischemia or infarction • Less when supplemental oxygen is used
Aortic valve stenosis	• Limited ability in increase cardiac output in response to hypotension from medications • Increased myocardial oxygen demand from left ventricular hypertrophy. Demand ischemia from hypotension or tachycardia
Dementia	• Increased sensitivity to sedatives • Delayed recovery • Paradoxical agitation is common (reversal agents may help) • Dose slowly and small
Pregnancy	• Aortocaval compression at 20 wk. 15° left uterine displacement • Benzodiazepines were once thought to cause cleft lip/palate. Probably not true. • Uteroplacental circulation and fetal well-being
Chronic pain	• Tolerance. May require very high narcotic dose • Naloxone contraindicated for oversedation

sedation by nonanesthesiologists to patients who are ASA class III or below. Furthermore, the Joint Commission may deem this an indication that the patient was assessed and found to be an appropriate candidate for the procedure and sedation. Second, those patients with significant comorbidities should have their disease processes maximally controlled prior to the administration of sedation. When appropriate, a multidisciplinary team approach should be employed, and consultation with an anesthesiologist should be considered. Finally, several disease processes place the patient at significant risk for complications from sedation (see Table 5.4). The pulmonary physician should use extreme caution when administering sedation to these patients.

Equipment and Monitoring

Bronchoscopy and other interventional pulmonary procedures are highly technical and require advanced equipment. In addition, the safe conduct of moderate or deep sedation requires that specific equipment be readily available, irrespective of the degree of complexity of the medical procedure. Table 5.5 describes the recommended equipment needed specifically for sedation.

Although the equipment outlined is important, the vigilance of a clinician monitoring the patient while under sedation is the most important factor influencing patient safety during moderate sedation. Inadequate monitoring of patients has been cited as both too common and a frequent cause of adverse events during bronchoscopy. The monitor, generally a nurse, should have no other significant clinical duties and must have the same training and privileging in the safe administration of sedation and rescue techniques as does the physician performing the procedure. The monitor should continuously evaluate the patient's respiratory rate, cardiac

Table 5.5. *Recommended equipment*

Category	Specific equipment
Airway	• Laryngoscopes: Multiple sizes • Endotracheal tubes: Multiple sizes with stylettes • Laryngeal airway mask • Oxygen source and appropriate tubing, masks, or nasal cannulae • Bag/mask ventilation device • Suction with appropriate suction device (Yankauer) • Oral and nasal airways: Multiple sizes
Monitoring	• Noninvasive blood pressure device • Electrocardiograph • Pulse oximeter • Capnograph (required for intubated patients)
Emergency	• Cardiac defibrillator • ACLS medications • Reversal agents (naloxone, flumazenil)
Intravenous access	• Gloves • Tourniquets • Alcohol wipes • IV catheters: Multiple sizes • IV tubing with needleless access ports • Tape • Appropriate IV fluids

Note: Adapted from Godwin SA, Caro DA, Wolf SJ, et al.

rate and rhythm, blood pressure, oxygen saturation, level of consciousness, and skin condition. These parameters should be documented every 5 minutes on a flow sheet designed specifically for moderate sedation (this document can be incorporated into the procedural documentation). In addition, the monitor should document the timing, dose, and indication for all medications administered and the amount of IV fluid administered. Recent literature has suggested the use of expiratory CO_2 monitoring as a way to objectively measure respiration.

Most of the physiologic parameters monitored during sedation are objective and relatively easy to measure. However, both the adequacy of respiration and the level of sedation can be more subjective and prone to error. Simply observing the rise and fall of the chest as a measure of respiration may be misleading as upper airway obstruction caused by oversedation does not prevent chest wall movement.

Thus, a patient may have no alveolar ventilation despite apparently normal chest wall movement. Even observing the presence of condensation on the oxygen mask during exhalation does not adequately assess minute ventilation or the presence of oversedation. Furthermore, the use of a full face mask is impractical during bronchoscopy. Given these limitations, the use of expired CO_2 monitors during moderate sedation has been recommended. This monitor identifies hypoventilation and patients at risk for hypoxemia before other clinical markers and with nearly 100% sensitivity. In one series, clinicians identified poor ventilation in only 3% of cases, whereas CO_2 monitoring found that 56% of patients were hypoventilated. More important, active intervention based on early detection of mild hypoventilation as indicated by expiratory CO_2 can effectively prevent subsequent hypoxia. Although measuring true end-tidal CO_2 may be impossible during bronchoscopy in a nonintubated patient, nasal cannula devices with side-port CO_2 detection may be used.

Monitoring the level of consciousness is fraught with subjectivity and inaccuracy. The definition of moderate sedation is that patients should respond to verbal commands, perhaps in conjunction with light touch. Furthermore, their protective reflexes should be intact. This standard is highly subjective, and is made more difficult when the protective airway reflexes are blunted by local anesthetics as is the case in bronchoscopy. Semiobjective scoring systems that monitor the patient's response to reproducible stimuli are often advocated, including the Ramsay score, the Continuum of Depth of Sedation Scale (CDSS), and the Observers Assessment of Alertness/Sedation Scale (OAAS). Each of these is based on a point scale, ranging from alert/anxious to unconscious. More recently, some authors have advocated the use of electroencephalogram- (EEG-) based physiologic monitoring to obtain more objective sedation data. This monitoring appears to correlate well with the Ramsay scale, OAAS, and CDSS. More importantly, it may allow clinicians to administer less medication and improve patient cooperation. More work needs to be done in this area before EEG-based monitors become standard sedation monitors.

Monitoring of the patient who has received moderate or deep sedation should continue in the postprocedure recovery area. Vital signs should be continually assessed and documented at regular intervals (generally every 1–30 minutes) while the patient is in the recovery area. Patients who received reversal agents (flumazenil or naloxone) should remain in the recovery area for at least 2 hours after the reversal is administered. For other patients, no predetermined recovery time should be required, but the patient should demonstrate objective evidence of recovery from the sedative medications prior to discharge to an in-patient unit or to home. Aldrete and Kroulik developed the postanesthesia recovery (PAR) scoring system, similar to the Apgar score for newborns, which helps to determine

readiness for discharge. This includes assigning 0–2 points for activity level, respiration, circulation consciousness, and oxygen saturation. (The original scoring system evaluated skin color, but this was modified when pulse oximetry became readily available.) When the patients reach a PAR score of 9 or 10, they are ready for discharge to the in-patient unit. Patients with a PAR score of 10 may still demonstrate significant impairment from the sedative medications, and thus a second level of assessment has been added to the PAR score to determine readiness for discharge home. This postanesthesia discharge (PAD) score includes assigning 0–2 points for the dressing, the level of pain, the ability to ambulate, the ability to drink liquids, and urine output. When the sum of the PAR and PAD scores is 18 or greater, the patient is ready for discharge. These scoring systems are used in dozens of countries and are accepted by The Joint Commission.

The medical center should develop specific discharge criteria based on the PAR and PAD score or other objective criteria. Independent licensed practitioners can then discharge patients in accordance with these criteria. Prior to final discharge home, patients and their families should be given verbal and written instructions regarding diet, level of activity and medications, and a 24-hour contact number in case of emergencies. All patients should be discharged in the presence of a responsible adult who will escort them home.

MEDICATIONS

Introduction

Moderate sedation represents a middle ground between the responsive and cooperative conditions of the lightly sedated patient and the unconscious, anesthetized condition of the patient under general anesthesia. Light sedation can always be augmented by the effective use of topical local anesthesia to numb the oropharynx and blunt the airway reflexes. During optimal situations, moderate sedation allows the patient to be

Table 5.6. *Common medications used in sedation and adult dosing schedules.*

Drug	Dose	Onset	Duration
Bolus type			
Midazolam	.5–2 mg	2 min	30 min
Fentanyl	25–100 μg	5 min	30 min
Ketorolac	15–30 mg	30 min	4–6 h
Infusion type			
Remifentanil	.1–.3 μg/kg/min	1–2 min	
Propofol	25–100 μg/kg/min	1–2 min	

comfortable, sleepy, amnestic, and stable hemo-dynamically with a modicum of medications. During difficult times, the patient is agitated, semiconscious, uncooperative, and tachycardic. Choosing the anesthetic medications to achieve optimal results requires an understanding of the kinetics and effects of each agent with its potential side effects and the patience to deliver divided doses and to titrate to effect. This section will review some of the commonly used medications in the delivery of moderate sedation to patients who are to undergo airway procedures. (See Table 5.6.)

Benzodiazepines

Midazolam is the most appropriate and commonly used benzodiazepine medication for moderate sedation. The combination of amnesia, anxiolysis, and sedation make midazolam an ideal drug either alone or in combination for moderate sedation during procedures that are of short duration and without significant painful stimulation. Midazolam may be administered IV, orally, intramuscularly, or rectally. Unlike the more lipid-soluble benzodiazepines lorazepam and diazepam, midazolam is not diluted in propylene glycol. This additive is associated with pain on injection and thrombophlebitis. In sedative doses, midazolam reaches peak effect in 2 minutes and produces sedation for 30 minutes. The rapid onset and short duration make midazolam a useful drug for moderate sedation by bolus injection or infusion.

All benzodiazepines act on the γ-aminobutyric acid (GABA) receptors by enhancing their affinity for GABA. The actions of GABA are to produce both sedation and anxiolysis [73]. Other drugs that act on GABA, such as barbiturates, etomidate, and propofol, can act synergistically to enhance the effects of the benzodiazepines. Other CNS depressants, such as opioids, anesthetic vapors, and α-2 agonists, also have synergistic effects when combined with a benzodiazepine.

Anterograde amnesia is an important component of all benzodiazepines. These agents produce amnestic effects that are out of proportion to the sedative effects. For example, patients may appear alert and conversant, but may remain amnestic for postoperative conversations and instructions. The condition is anterograde (not retrograde) amnesia, and this distinction is frequently misstated. Although the event that is forgotten has occurred in the past, the storage of that event in a patient's memory happens after the administration of midazolam, and thus is properly termed anterograde amnesia. Benzodiazepine cannot reliably cause patients to forget events that occurred before the medication was administered.

Midazolam should be used with caution in elderly patients or in patients with impaired liver function. Midazolam is highly protein bound and is cleared by the liver; therefore, patients with decreased concentrations of serum albumin or with decreased cytochrome P-450 enzymatic activity will have exaggerated effects and duration of activity. Agents that either raise or lower the cytochrome P-450 activity will also affect the action of midazolam. Sedative doses should be administered in a divided fashion, leaving sufficient time to assess the clinical effect of each interval dose. Midazolam does have a reversal agent, flumazenil, which will be discussed later.

Opioids

Although the opioid class of drugs includes dozens of medications with natural and synthetic origins, the major differences consist of their potencies and their rates of equilibration. All opioids are μ-receptor agonists, and this action accounts for their analgesic properties. In addition to the desired analgesic and antitussive effects, all μ-agonists share the side effects of nausea, vomiting, itching, muscle rigidity, and respiratory depression. The use of preemptive antiemetics has been shown to prevent the nausea and vomiting caused by opioids. Fentanyl has been shown to cause chest wall muscular rigidity more often than other synthetic opioids. In some cases, the chest wall rigidity is so severe that it can compromise ventilation and can only be successfully treated with the administration of neuromuscular blocking agents (paralytics). To be effective for moderate sedation, opioids should have high potency and rapidly reach equilibration. Fentanyl and remifentanil possess these properties.

Fentanyl is highly protein bound, lipid soluble, and metabolized by the liver. The time to peak analgesic effect following a single IV bolus is 5 minutes. The lipid solubility facilitates the movement of fentanyl across the blood–brain barrier. A single dose will last 30 minutes. Much of the initial bolus is taken up by inactive tissue sites in the lung, fat, and skeletal muscle. As these tissue sites become saturated by either repeated doses or by a continuous infusion, the context-sensitive half-life becomes longer. With continued administration of fentanyl, the half-life approaches the elimination half-life of 3–4

hours. Therefore, the advantage of fentanyl as a short-acting agent is lessened as the duration of the procedure requires multiple repeated boluses or a continuous infusion. Specific opioid antagonists do exist and will be discussed later.

An alternative opioid to fentanyl that can be used for both brief procedures and those with varying duration is remifentanil. This opioid is used for general anesthesia only, as remifentanil will cause apnea. Remifentanil is a synthetic opioid with equivalent potency to fentanyl; both are about 100 times more potent than morphine. A rapid onset of analgesic effect occurs after an IV bolus of remifentanil, with peak effect within 1–1.5 minutes. Unlike the other synthetic opioids, remifentanil has a unique degradation, being metabolized by plasma esterases. The elimination half-life is 8–20 minutes and is independent of liver or kidney function. Repeated dosing or continuous infusions do not prolong the elimination half-life. For example, a 5-hour infusion of remifentanil produced return of breathing within 3–5 minutes following discontinuation. Rapid elimination of remifentanil means that it does not provide any residual analgesia in the postoperative period. Other analgesics need to be started in the recovery area.

It is important to realize that all opioids have the unique property of providing intense pain relief without loss of proprioception or consciousness. Although this property has brought comfort to millions, it also brings the possibility of awareness. Intraoperative awareness under general anesthesia is a recognized complication and one that is more common when opioids are used. Awareness during moderate sedation should be an expected condition, but often patients will complain of hearing and feeling portions of their procedure. It is essential that anyone who is planning to administer moderate sedation advise the patient that some degree of recall is to be expected.

Propofol

Under the general heading of sedatives/hypnotics, propofol emerges as a versatile and effective agent to use when administering moderate sedation. Currently the most commonly used parenteral anesthetic agent in the United States, propofol is a substituted isopropylphenol that is insoluble in water and usually prepared in a lipid vehicle for IV administration. The emulsion consists of soybean oil, egg lecithin, and glycerol. Disodium ethylene diamine tetraacetic acid (EDTA) or sodium metabisulfite is added as a preservative and to inhibit bacterial growth, but the propofol mixture does support bacterial proliferation and serious infections have been reported.

As with the benzodiazepines and other sedatives/hypnotics, propofol acts on the GABA receptors and decreases the dissociation rate of GABA from the receptor. Metabolized in the liver by cytochrome P-450, there is also extensive nonhepatic metabolism as well as inactive tissue uptake. As a result of these elimination pathways, the context-sensitive half-life is not prolonged in such conditions as a propofol infusion lasting 8 hours. Propofol concentrations are not elevated in cirrhotic or alcoholic patients (suggesting the ability of the extrahepatic pathways to metabolize propofol) nor in patients with renal failure, but concentrations are higher in elderly patients.

Propofol produces rapid sedation without associated nausea or vomiting and a rapid return of cognitive function. Either an infusion or incremental boluses every 5 minutes can create levels of moderate sedation. The potential side effects of propofol include hypotension, apnea, and airway obstruction, so the patient needs to have close hemodynamic monitoring and immediate access to emergency airway interventions. Propofol does not seem to provoke bronchospasm. It often produces pain at the injection site, but this pain incidence can be reduced to <10% with the administration into a large vein (e.g., antecubital) or pretreatment with 1% lidocaine or opioids. The use of propofol by health care providers other than anesthetists is controversial. Many states require that the providers be certified in sedation techniques and competent in managing the airway.

Severe lactic acidosis as a consequence of prolonged propofol administration has been described in both adults and children. Although initially described with propofol infusions lasting more than 24 hours, there have been a number of reports of acidosis developing in shorter durations. Any patient on a propofol infusion with an unexplained tachycardia should be suspected of having "propofol infusion syndrome." The arterial blood gas and serum lactate levels should indicate a metabolic acidosis. Other causes of metabolic acidosis – such as tourniquet release, diabetic ketoacidosis, sepsis, and hyperchloremic metabolic acidosis from extensive infusions of normal saline – should be excluded. Treatment includes discontinuation of the propofol and supportive care, which has included extracorporeal membrane oxygenation in at least one report. The mechanism for propofol infusion syndrome appears to be interruption of the electron transport chain and impairment of the long-chain fatty acid metabolism.

Nonsteroidal Antiinflammatory Drugs (NSAIDs)

The NSAIDs share the three properties of acting as analgesics, antiinflammatories, and antipyretics. Although a larger, heterogeneous group of medications exists in this category, ketorolac is the only applicable drug to the administration of moderate sedation. As one of the few NSAIDs approved for parenteral use, ketorolac has greater analgesic activity than antiinflammatory activity. As a traditional NSAID, ketorolac does block cyclooxygenase-1 and therefore does promote gastric ulceration and platelet inhibition.

Administered as a sole analgesic or in combination with opioids to potentiate the analgesic effect, ketorolac provides rapid pain relief. Ketorolac does not induce tolerance nor does it cause respiratory depression. In patients with an aspirin allergy, nasal polyposis, or asthma, ketorolac has been reported to trigger life-threatening bronchospasm. Patients with congestive heart failure, hypovolemia, or hepatorenal syndrome may be susceptible to ketorolac-induced renal failure because of their dependence on local renal prostaglandin production to maintain renal blood flow.

Antiemetics

The sensation of nausea and act of emesis are a coordinated set of muscular, autonomic, behavioral, and emotional responses that exist to rid the stomach of toxins. In clinical practice, nausea and vomiting are unpleasant and unintended consequences to anesthesia, inflammation, or motion that can add morbidity to and complicate the recovery from any procedure. The coordination of the vomiting response occurs in the central emesis center in the lateral reticular formation of the mid brainstem in the area adjacent to both the chemoreceptor trigger zone (CTZ), found in the area postrema at the base of the fourth ventricle, and the nucleus solitarius of the vagal nerve. The CTZ monitors the cerebrospinal fluid for toxins and receives information from the gut. The emesis center also receives information from the cerebral cortex regarding anticipatory nausea and vestibular input with respect to motion sickness.

This complex neural connection has a variety of neurotransmitter influences. Serotonin, histamine, acetylcholine, dopamine, and prostaglandins have key roles in the neural modulation of the emesis center. The antiemetic strategy, therefore, can be targeted at one or several of these neural modulators. For example, ondansetron can block the specific 5-hydroxytryptamine—3 receptors in the CTZ, and the antihistamine cyclizine or the antimuscarinic scopolamine can block the vestibular input from motion sickness. A steroid such as dexamethasone can block the emetogenic influence from inflammation, and benzodiazepines can suppress anticipatory nausea. Therefore, the cause of the nausea may differ in different patients, and the effective treatment may address the particular etiology. Often, however, multiple medications that use a variety of mechanisms of action are required to reduce the symptoms of nausea and prevent vomiting.

Ondansetron is structurally similar to serotonin, and an IV dose reaches peak effect within 30–60 minutes. Interestingly, the drug conveys antiemetic action long after it has disappeared from the plasma circulation, suggesting a continued interaction at the serotonin receptor. For this reason, all the serotonin antagonists may be given once daily. Metabolized in the liver by cytochrome P-450 enzymes, ondansetron should be reduced in patients with liver failure, although no such reduction is needed in elderly patients. Ondansetron is effective for nausea from chemotherapy and postoperative sources but is ineffective in treating motion sickness. Side effects from ondansetron are usually headache and diarrhea. The usual dose of ondansetron in the postoperative setting is 4 mg IV. Higher doses do not show greater reduction of postoperative nausea and vomiting.

Reversal Agents

All medication antagonists have their own chemical properties, kinetics, binding characteristics, and elimination pathways. The constellation of characteristics will determine how well the antagonist can reverse the action of the agonist, but also will determine what other concerns the practitioner should have in the process of using a reversal agent.

An imidazolebenzodiazepine, flumazenil binds with high affinity to sites on the GABA-A receptor. Flumazenil, when combined with a benzodiazepine, does not produce water. In other words, all drugs have side effects, and using one to reverse the effects of another does not come without some risk. Flumazenil competitively inhibits the binding of both agonists and reverse agonists to the GABA-A receptor. Slight activity, which resembles a reverse agonist at low concentrations and an agonist at high concentrations, has been reported. The agonist activity of flumazenil, however, does not prevent the withdrawal symptoms that have been reported. Just as withdrawal from chronic benzodiazepine use can cause a variety of effects, flumazenil can cause dysphoria, irritability, anorexia, sweating tremors, unpleasant dreams, dizziness, exacerbation of insomnia or anxiety, and frank seizures. Flumazenil is not recommended in patients who are taking antiseizure medication.

Usually, 1–5 mg of flumazenil is given in divided doses between 1 and 10 minutes until the desired reversal of sedation is achieved. The clinical effects last from 30 to 60 minutes and, therefore, the potential for resedation is possible and the flumazenil may need to be rebolused or an infusion started. If 5 mg of flumazenil does not reverse sedation, the sedation was probably not caused by benzodiazepine overdose. In practice, benzodiazepine overdose rarely causes respiratory depression, and, therefore, the urgent need for reversal using flumazenil is exceedingly uncommon.

As with flumazenil, the administration of naloxone to reverse the effects of opioids does not produce water. A nonselective competitive antagonist, naloxone binds with high affinity to all three opioid receptors (μ, Δ, κ). Used to treat narcotic-induced depression of ventilation, the side effect of naloxone is to also reverse narcotic-induced analgesia. Postsurgical patients can develop hyperacute, severe pain. The activation of the sympathetic nervous system in response to naloxone-induced pain can include tachycardia, hypertension, pulmonary edema, and cardiac arrhythmias, including ventricular fibrillation. Plasma cortisol and catecholamine levels rise following naloxone administration. Less obvious side effects from naloxone are decreased performance on memory tests and dysphoria.

Given in divided doses of 1–4 µg/kg, naloxone quickly reverses opioid-induced respiratory depression and has a short duration of action (30–45 minutes). Thus, the effects of naloxone may be shorter than the half-life of the opioid that is causing the respiratory depression. A continuous infusion of naloxone may be necessary and is usually started at 5 (µg/kg)/h.

In clinical practice, careful titration of the opioid medications with understanding of the time to peak activity and the potential for respiratory depression should make the use of opioid antagonists uncommon. Opioid doses should be adjusted in elderly patients and in patients with limited hepatic function or poor pulmonary reserve. Opioid doses should be adjusted downward whenever other sedative agents are used in combination. Finally, the narcotic effect should be reserved with naloxone as a rescue strategy when respiratory depression occurs and when mechanical or supplemental breathing measures are not practical or beneficial in improving the situation.

COMPLICATIONS OF SEDATION

Complications from moderate sedation can occur, from undersedation, oversedation, and idiosyncratic responses to "therapeutic levels" of sedation. Too little sedation can lead to excessive movement, delirium, and pain. Too much sedation can produce hemodynamic collapse and respiratory depression. Even those patients receiving "optimal" therapeutic concentrations of sedation can demonstrate allergic reactions, rigidity, or laryngospasm. Even therapeutic levels of sedatives can worsen such conditions as acute intermittent porphyria, malignant hyperthermia, or carcinoid crisis. Specific complications can occur with specific pharmacologic agents, such as adrenal suppression from etomidate and rhabdomyolysis from propofol. This section will focus on the general complications that occur from oversedation.

Most sedatives are myocardial depressants and/or vasodilators that can act to profoundly lower blood pressure. The degree of cardiovascular depression will depend on the patient's cardiovascular and volume status, any medications that have additive effects on the blood pressure, and any surgical conditions that may affect the patient. For example, the reverse Trendelenburg position can lower the preload and cause an exaggerated hypotensive response to sedatives. Effects on the blood pressure from sedation can be greater in patients with cardiomyopathy, valvular heart disease, or pericardial conditions, such as acute tamponade. Resuscitative drugs should always be immediately available to administer when a sedative is given.

Many sedatives are respiratory depressants and, in large enough doses, can cause apnea. Most sedatives blunt the ventilatory response to both high levels of carbon dioxide and low levels of oxygen. For this reason, all patients who receive sedation need to be monitored for both ventilation and oxygenation. Respiratory rates can be misleading, however, as they may not reflect minute ventilation. For this reason, either minute ventilation or end-tidal CO_2 should be used for deeper sedation techniques, to better detect hypoventilation. For oxygenation status, the pulse oximeter provides a reliable and sensitive predictor of desaturation in most settings. Evidence of hypoxemia may not occur until the patient has been hypoventilating or apneic for several minutes. To rescue patients from conditions of hypoventilation or hypoxemia, advanced airway equipment needs to be immediately available, along with a source of enriched oxygen, continuous suction, and the trained personnel to use them.

In conclusion, the use of moderate sedation to allow the accomplishment of airway procedures requires a balance of anesthetic drugs with their relaxant, sedative, and analgesic effects with the unwanted and potentially dangerous side effects. The conduct of the anesthetic and the recognition of these side effects require planning and monitoring. Every patient needs a history and physical examination, including an examination of the airway. All patients need standard monitoring and a person designated as the monitor. Each bronchoscopic procedure requires the proper equipment, medications, and training to administer the medications and to deal with side effects. Finally, all patients need a safe environment in which to recover from sedation. With careful preparation, proper supplies, and protocols, bronchoscopy can be performed under excellent surgical conditions and with minimal adverse events.

SUGGESTED READINGS

Aldrete JA. Post-anesthetic recovery score. *J Am Coll Surg.* 2007;205:e3–e4.

Aldrete JA, Kroulik D. A postanesthetic recovery score. *Anesth Analg.* 1970;49:924–934.

Bahhady IJ, Ernst A. Risks of and recommendations for flexible bronchoscopy in pregnancy: a review. *Chest.* 2004;126:1974–1981.

British Thoracic Society guidelines on diagnostic flexible bronchoscopy. *Thorax.* 2001;56(Suppl):i11–i2l.

Burton JH, Harrah JD, Germann CA, Dillon DC. Does end-tidal carbon dioxide monitoring detect respiratory events prior to current sedation monitoring practices? *Acad Emerg Med.* 2006;13:500–504.

Chisholm CJ, Zurica J, Mironov D, et al. Comparison of electrophysiologic monitors with clinical assessment of level of sedation. *Mayo Clin Proc.* 2006;81:46–52.

Day RO, Chalmers DRC, Williams KM, Campbell TJ. Death of a healthy volunteer in a human research project: implications for Australian clinical research. *Med J Aust.* 1998;168:449–451.

Doenicke AW, Roizen MF, Rau J, et al. Pharmacokinetics and pharmacodynamics of propofol in a new solvent. *Anesth Analg.* 1997;85:1399–1403.

Fudickar A, Bein B, Tonner PH. Propofol infusion syndrome in anaesthesia and intensive care medicine. *Curr Opin Anaesthesiol.* 2006;19;404–410.

Godwin SA, Caro DA, Wolf SJ, et al. Clinical policy: procedural sedation and analgesia in the emergency department. *Ann Emerg Med.* 2005;45:177–196.

Hatton MQF, Allen MB, Vathenen AS, et al. Does sedation help in fiberoptic bronchoscopy? *BMJ.* 1994;309:1206–1207.

Honeybourne D, Neumann CS. An audit of bronchoscopy practice in the United Kingdom: a survey of adherence to national guidelines. *Thorax.* 1997; 52:709–713.

Hwang JCF, Hanowell LH, Mott JM, et al. Perioperative bronchoscopy. In: Hanowell LH, Waldron RJ, eds. *Airway Management.* Philadelphia: Lippincott-Raven; 1996.

Isaac PA, Barry JE, Vaughan RS, et al. A jet nebulizer for delivery of topical anesthesia to the respiratory tract: a comparison with cricothyroid puncture and direct spraying for fiberoptic bronchoscopy. *Anaesthesia.* 1990;45:46–48.

The Joint Commission. Pre-induction assessment for sedation and analgesia. Available at: http://www.jointcommission.org/AccreditationPrograms/Hospitals/

Standards/FAQs/Provision+of+Care/Assessment/Pre_Induction.htm. Accessed November 29, 2007.

Jones DA, McBurney A, Stanley PJ, et al. Plasma concentrations of lignocaine and its metabolites during fiberoptic bronchoscopy. *Br J Anaesth*. 1982;54:853–857.

Kane GC, Hoehn SM, Behrenbeck TR, Mulvagh SL. Benzocaine-induced methemoglobinemia based on the Mayo Clinic experience from 28,478 transesophageal echocardiograms: incidence, outcomes, and predisposing factors. *Arch Intern Med*. 2007;167:1977–1982.

Kimura T, Watanabe S, Asakura N, et al. Determination of end-tidal sevoflurane concentration for tracheal intubation and minimum alveolar anesthetic concentration in adults. *Anesth Analg*. 1994;79:3780–3781.

Lundgren R, Haggmark S, Reiz S. Hemodynamic effects of flexible fiberoptic bronchoscopy performed under topical anesthesia. *Chest*. 1982;82:295–299.

Matot I, Kramer MR. Sedation in outpatient bronchoscopy. *Respir Med*. 2000;94:1145–1153.

Matot I, Kramer MR, Glantz L, et al. Myocardial ischemia in sedated patients undergoing fiberoptic bronchoscopy. *Chest*. 1997;112:1454–1458.

Makaryus JN, Makaryus AN, Johnson M. Acute myocardial infarction following the use of intranasal anesthetic cocaine. *South Med J*. 2006;99:79–61.

Middleton RM, Shah A, Kirkpatrick MB. Topical nasal anesthesia for flexible bronchoscopy. A comparison of four methods in normal subjects and in patients undergoing transnasal bronchoscopy. *Chest*. 1991;99:1093–1096.

Mulroy MF. Peripheral nerve blockade. In: Barash PG, Cullen BF, Stoelting RK, eds. *Clinical Anesthesia, 2nd ed*. Philadelphia: Lippincott Williams & Wilkins; 1992.

Osula S, Stockton P, Adbelaziz MM, Walshaw MJ. Intratracheal cocaine induced myocardial infarction: an unusual complication of fiberoptic bronchoscopy. *Thorax*. 2003;58:733–734.

Parker MRJ, Day CJE, Coote AH. Sedation in fiberoptic bronchoscopy. *BMJ*. 1995;310:872.

Ramsay MAE, Savege TM, Simpson BRI, Goodwin R. Controlled sedation with alphaxolone-alphadolone. *BMJ*. 1974;ii:656–658.

Reed AP. Preparation of the patient for awake flexible fiberoptic bronchoscopy. *Chest*. 1992;101:244–253.

Riker RR, Picard JT, Fraser GL. Prospective evaluation of the Sedation-Agitation Score for adult critically ill patients. *Crit Care Med*. 1999;27:1325–1329.

Schreiber F. Austrian Society of Gastroenterology and Hepatology–Guideline on sedation and monitoring during gastrointestinal endoscopy. *Endoscopy*. 2007;39:259–262.

Simpson FG, Arnold AG, Purvis A, et al. Postal survey of bronchoscopy practice by physicians in the United Kingdom. *Thorax*. 1986;41:311–317.

Smith CM, Stead RJ. Survey of flexible fiberoptic bronchoscopy in the United Kingdom. *Eur Respir J*. 2002;19:458–463.

Stoelting K, Hillier S, eds. *Pharmacology & Physiology in Anesthetic Practice*. Philadelphia: Lippincott Williams & Wilkins; 2006.

Stolz D, Chhajed PN, Leuppi J, et al. Nebulized lidocaine for flexible bronchoscopy: a randomized, double-blind, placebo-controlled trial. *Chest*. 2005;128:1756–1760.

Villegas T. Sleep apnea and moderate sedation. *Gastroenterol Nurs*. 2004;27:121–124.

Weaver CS, Hauter WH, Duncan CE, et al. An assessment of the association of bispectral index with 2 clinical sedation scales for monitoring depth of procedural sedation. *Am J Emerg Med*. 2007;25:918–924.

Williams KA, Barker GL, Harwood RJ, Woodall NM. Combined nebulization and spray-as-you-go topical local anaesthesia of the airway. *Br J Anaesth*. 2005;95:549–553.

Wolf A, Weir P, Setage P, et al. Impaired fatty acid oxidation in propofol infusion syndrome. *Lancet*. 2001;357:606–607.

6

ANATOMY AND CARE OF THE BRONCHOSCOPE

Robert Garland

The flexible bronchoscope has undergone many technological advances since it was first introduced more than 40 years ago [1]. But, despite these advances in imaging and ease of use, it remains a fragile piece of equipment and susceptible to damage [2]. If improvements can be made to the quality of the image and the size of the working channel without compromising the overall diameter of the instrument, why can't significant improvements be made to the durability of the bronchoscope? Very simply put, there is so much technology stuffed into such a small compartment that even slight trauma to the instrument can be devastating.

It is truly remarkable that this equipment can perform all the functions that it does when you consider the difficulties in engineering such a small diameter instrument. Let's consider the challenges we must overcome in developing the flexible bronchoscopes that are available today.

CHALLENGES AND BASIC REQUIREMENTS OF THE BRONCHOSCOPE

The bronchoscope must accomplish several feats with some challenging obstacles that it must overcome:

■ It must be small enough to fit into the airway and still provide space for breathing.

■ The airway does not have any illumination, so we must provide artificial light to see where we are going.

■ There are bifurcations in the airway, so we need a mechanism for steering the instrument.

■ The airway can be obstructed with fluid or blood, so we must have a way to clear those to continue our journey.

■ We need a way to take samples of the airway should we see something abnormal.

■ It may be beneficial if we could document a finding to share with others by capturing an image of it.

ANATOMY AND PHYSIOLOGY OF THE BRONCHOSCOPE

Now that we have identified the needs of the bronchoscope, let's take a look at how the current bronchoscopes accomplish this. I would like to distinguish between the anatomy (structure) and the physiology (function) of the instrument (Figure 6.1).

Anatomy

The bronchoscope is designed to be held in the left hand because the universal cord (the part of the scope that plugs into the light source) comes off the left side of the control section of the scope, and the weight of the scope is supported by this hand. There are three basic components to the flexible bronchoscope [3]:

- Control section
- Insertion tube
- Universal cord

Control Section

This is the part of the bronchoscope that you hold with your left hand. This part is designed so that the operator can perform multiple functions with this hand while still gripping the scope (the right hand should only be used to hold the insertion tube at the area closest to where it enters the patient).

There is a lever that can be moved up or down by the thumb that controls the angle of the distal tip for steering and a valve that can be compressed by the first finger to control the vacuum applied to the airways. Most scopes available today have a separate valve on the control section that allows for placement of accessories for sampling the airway.

Also on the control section is a series of remote switches that can be programmed for a variety of functions such as capturing images, magnifying the field, and even applying different wavelengths of light to the airways.

Insertion Tube

This is the section of the instrument that actually enters the patient and consists of a flexible catheter, which in the adult bronchoscope is between 55 and 60 mm and usually has an outer diameter of between 5 and 6 cm in length. Depending on the size of the outer diameter, there is a plastic catheter between 2 and 3 mm traveling through the middle of the insertion tube that is used for passing accessories or sampling fluid or tissue. This is known as the working channel.

Running alongside the catheter are two fiber-optic bundles that carry light from an external light source to provide illumination to the airways where no natural light can reach. There are

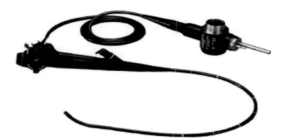

FIGURE 6.1. Flexible bronchoscope.

two thin wires that are connected to a lever in the control body, pass through the insertion tube, and connect at the distal end of the scope to a series of hinged devices that are used for steering the instrument. Whether the scope's imaging system is considered fiber-optic or video chip technology, there are either fiber bundles or several electrical wires that transmit an electronic image through this insertion tube after receiving the image from a small lens at the distal end of the scope. All of these delicate catheters, fibers, cables, and wires are wrapped with a flexible but strong metal sheath to protect them somewhat from the potential damage of human teeth and user error. Outside of this sheath a thin, waterproof membrane is applied to separate the devastating effects of moisture from the internal components.

Universal Cord

This section of the bronchoscope carries information and light to and from the control body, the video processor, and the light source. At one end is a connector that attaches to the external light source and video processor, and the other end provides a support for the hand that holds the instrument as it is permanently connected to the control body.

Physiology

The primary function of the bronchoscope is to provide an inspection of the airways. To accomplish this, many components of the equipment need to work together. I like to think of the function of the scope as a series of independent systems that rely on one another for the smooth

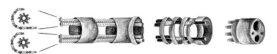

FIGURE 6.3. Mechanical system.

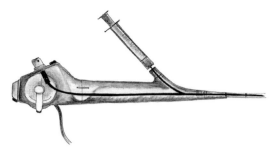

FIGURE 6.2. Plumbing system.

operation of the instrument. There are four systems that make up the bronchoscope as we know it today [3].

Plumbing System

The working channel acts as a conduit for passing accessory instruments for sampling the airways and also as a channel to remove secretions and blood to allow proper viewing. In most bronchoscopes there are two ways to access the working channel. At the top of the control section there is a valve that, when compressed, allows communication between the working channel and a vacuum source that has been attached to the valve. This then applies suction to the channel and clears whatever fluid is in front of the scope. There is usually a second valve on the control section that accessory devices or fluid can be placed through to allow sampling of the lung. This valve works by having a narrow opening in the housing that will close when nothing is in it and will open only enough for the device to pass through. This allows the operator to apply suction even though the channel is partially obstructed with the device. These valves snap on to a seat in the control section and are usually considered single-use items as they are difficult to properly clean (Figure 6.2).

Mechanical System

A series of levers, wires, and hinged metal bands make up the parts of the mechanical system that allow the operator to "steer" his or her instrument to specific locations in the airways. As described above, there is a lever on the control

section that can be moved up or down by the thumb that in turn pulls or pushes thin wires running through the insertion tube to the bending section of the scope at the distal tip, which moves this hinged section anterior or posterior relative to the orientation of the scope. This system is similar to the "chain and sprocket system" used to move bicycles. The amount of "angulation" varies depending on the scope but is usually around 180° up and 130° down. Over time, the wires can become stretched and the angulation will become less, and adjustments will need to be made to bring it back to specifications (Figure 6.3).

Electrical System

This system serves many functions in the modern bronchoscope that most of us take for granted. In the video bronchoscope that is commonly used today, the electrical system helps to carry the signals from the video chip to the video processor to be converted to an image that we then understand. It also allows the operator with a press of his or her finger to perform functions on the remote switches like capturing images, magnifying the image, or altering the light to which the tissue is exposed.

One of the most important features is that it provides the feedback from the processor to allow for corrections in areas like light intensity. There is a difference in the light needed to illuminate the airway depending on how close the end of the lens is to the tissue and whether there are secretions in the field reflecting the light. This feedback will reduce the amount of light if the area under inspection is very close to the tissue or if there is excessive reflection from fluid or secretions (Figure 6.4).

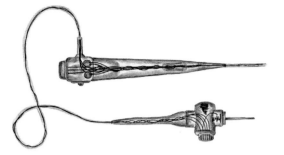

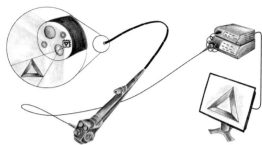

FIGURE 6.4. Electrical system.

FIGURE 6.5. Imaging system with monitor.

Image System

The quality of imaging is truly amazing in the instruments that are in use today, especially when you stop to consider that you may be seeing images on a 19-inch video monitor with the clarity of almost high definition taken from a lens that is only a little more than 1 mm wide. To be able to see deep into a body cavity with this clarity poses many challenges. First, we must provide enough light through a tube that has to be small enough to pass through the adult vocal cords; this requires that the whole tube cannot be much more than 6 mm in diameter. Then we must remember that some of the passages turn back on themselves, so the scope must be able to bend completely 180° without kinking and damaging its components (Figure 6.5).

How do we get by all of these obstacles?

First, the airway is illuminated by an external light source that is attached to the bronchoscope. The light is carried through the scope via a series of glass fibers wrapped tightly in a bundle that allows the light to bend around corners. There are two fiber bundles needed to provide enough light to the distal end of the scope so that the light is distributed evenly without it looking like one is shining a flashlight down the airway. This prevents a bright spot in the middle of the field while the edges are progressively dimmer. If one of these fiber bundles is damaged, then you may see an area of brighter concentration of light in one part of the airway.

The very end of the bronchoscope contains a tiny lens that magnifies and focuses the image either on the fiber bundle in a fiber-optic scope or on a video chip in a video system. In the fiber-optic scope, the image is carried through this fiber bundle to another lens that magnifies and refocuses it. In the later video systems, the image is disassembled into light levels and colors and sent up a series of wires, where it is reassembled into an image in the video processor.

Given that we are viewing this image from a lens that is 1 mm wide, it is remarkable that we have a field of view of 120°. Most of the scopes today have the ability to view the image at a depth of between 3 and 100 mm, so this allows the operator to be very close to the object in question, and is necessary when working in an airway that is 10–20 mm wide. It is also important to remember that, as we view the image on a monitor, any accessories passed through it will appear at 3 o'clock from the center of the image (Figure 6.5).

TYPES OF BRONCHOSCOPES AVAILABLE

All bronchoscopes that are available to the user today use the systems that we discussed earlier; they just use different technologies to accomplish the same thing. It is important to remember that there are compromises that are made when one wants to (for instance) have an image superior to that of another scope of the same size.

Because there is a relatively fixed outer diameter that can be used for the insertion tube, any space used to occupy the technology to improve the image will leave less space for the other functions of the scope. Therefore, the instrument that gives you improved imaging may not be able to offer the size of (for instance) a working channel that is the best available on the market. Here are some examples of the categories of bronchoscopes available to the user today.

Nonvideo

These original bronchoscopes were far different than the instruments available to users today. The light and images were transmitted via a series of glass fibers called fiber-optic bundles. This technology allowed for the flexible bronchoscope to come to be, as prior to this development there was no way to allow light to "bend" as is required with the flexible bronchoscope.

The bronchoscope had a lens at either end of the instrument that allowed the operator to view the airway by looking directly through the eyepiece. The lens at the distal end of the scope (objective lens) would create and focus the image for its travel up the insertion tube (via thousands of glass fibers, called the fiber-optic bundle) to the eyepiece lens, where the image was then magnified and refocused to the user's desire.

The image from a nonvideo scope can be viewed on the monitor of a video system with the use of a video converter: One end attaches to the eyepiece of the nonvideo scope, and the other end attaches to the video processor. The image can then be viewed by others besides the operator, but this image is inferior to that of the true video system.

Video

The video bronchoscope was a significant improvement in endoscopic technology by providing better imaging with the use of the charge-coupled device (CCD) chip. This chip, placed directly behind the objective lens, eliminates the fiber-optic bundle. Even though it has the advantage of allowing light to bend, the fiber-optic bundle was no comparison to the CCD chip in

the way images can be transmitted. The chip converts the image (as is seen through the objective lens) into electronic signals that are carried via wires to the video processor for reassembly into an image that can be understood by the human eye.

There were many other developments that occurred because of the integration of the bronchoscope and the video processor (white balance, zoom). These developments will be discussed later in this chapter.

Hybrid

Because of space limitations with some equipment, some of the bronchoscopes available in the market today are a combination of the materials that make up the video and nonvideo instruments. An example would be a small-diameter bronchoscope, the size of which may be necessary for navigating in distal airways and which has superior imaging that would not be available with the nonvideo scope. The insertion tube (because of its narrow diameter requirements) may not be able to "accept" the size of a CCD chip, so the older fiber-optic bundle may have to be used to transmit imaging through the insertion tube to a point in the control section where a CCD chip could be placed to perform the function of transmitting image technology via an electronic signal to the video processor. The advantage is improved imaging over a true fiber-optic system.

THE VIDEO PROCESSOR

The primary purpose of the video processor is of course to process the electrical signals that were produced by the video chip in the bronchoscope so that they can be read by the video monitor. That unto itself is quite a feat, but there are hosts of other "behind the scenes" functions that happen inside this little box. Some are manual functions that the operator has control over, and others are done based on feedback that the processor has interpreted as needing adjustment [4].

Some manual adjustments are as follows:

- White balance control: This function, which should be performed before each procedure, adjusts the color that was created by the video chip to accommodate the color of the light source . . . in other words, it teaches the processor to understand that the color white is really white.
- Image color adjustment: This allows fine tuning of the colors but should be made only after the white balance function is performed.
- Iris settings: This is a manual adjustment that is usually used in the "average" mode, but can be changed to "peak" mode to view areas that appear washed out.
- Image enhancement: This gives the operator the ability to enhance the image to meet his or her needs.

Some automatic adjustments include:

- Auto-focus: Depending on the depth of the field, the system adjusts for the distance to the object to provide focusing without manual adjustments.
- Automatic brightness control: This automatically adjusts the light to the airway to maintain a constant level of brightness even if the distance changes from the end of the scope to the object being viewed.

Other options that an operator has control over through the video processor controls are:

- Video freeze, capture, enlargement, picture in picture, and other programming
- The ability to access scope history; the number of uses, and scope serial number
- The ability to save images to a video capture card in the event that there is not a computer or printer attached

INTEGRATION OF THE BRONCHOSCOPE WITH OTHER COMPONENTS OF THE SYSTEM TO CREATE THE VIDEO SYSTEM

Correct integration of the flexible bronchoscope with the other components of the bronchoscopy system is critical to proper visualization of the image and can not be taken lightly. The operators need to ensure that the system is functioning properly prior to the examination and, whether they rely on their own internal support or an outside department (such as clinical engineering), there needs to be a system in place to correct for any issues that may arise during a procedure during which one cannot afford to lose an image at a critical time. Refer to manufacturer's instruction manual for specific applications.

There are many configurations that one can use to route the image from the bronchoscope to the video monitor, but generally the information flows from the camera in the bronchoscope through the video processor to the video monitor [5]. Peripherals such as video recorders can get their feeds either before or after the monitor. The way the image is transmitted to the video monitor depends on the outputs in the video processor, but can include a variety of sources such as composite, super video (S-video); red, green, blue (RGB), or (in some later processors) serial digital interface/digital video interface (SDI/DVI). It is critical for the operator to realize that the quality of the image on the monitor is only as good as its weakest link. In other words, you may be spending unnecessary money for a high-definition monitor if your cameras (i.e., bronchoscopes) are not of similar quality.

PROPER CARE OF THE FLEXIBLE BRONCHOSCOPE

This section is by far the most important part of this chapter. The average bronchoscope has almost doubled in price over the last 10 years, and today costs well over $20,000. We must remember that this equipment is not only expensive to purchase, it is also very expensive to repair. In a busy program, the cost of repairs can exceed $100,000 per year; many of these repairs can be prevented [6]. One of the best ways to prevent damage is to read and follow the instruction manual for each instrument.

The intention of this book is to introduce basic bronchoscopy procedures, so procedures that fall under the category of interventional pulmonology will not be discussed here [7].

To keep with a systematic approach to the care of the bronchoscope, I have divided this section into three parts to distinguish between how to care for the equipment during different aspects of the bronchoscopy procedure [8,9]. These sections will be grouped as preprocedure, intraprocedure, and postprocedure.

Preprocedure Care of the Bronchoscope

Items to consider before the procedure will include:

A. Transportation of the instrument to the procedure area: Transport the scope from the storage area to the bronchoscopy suite in something that will protect it from damage and dust (i.e., a plastic bin that is covered on the top)
B. A preprocedure check of the systems
   1. Plumbing: Do the valves work and are channels clear?
   2. Mechanical: Does the bending section flex the proper amount and in the right direction?
   3. Electrical: Are all power systems functioning: processor, light source, and monitor?
   4. Image: Do you get a crisp image with good color?
C. Proper preparation for the operator
   1. Proper lubrication of scope: Oil-based lubricants can degrade the rubber sheath; water-based lubricants are recommended.
   2. Make sure that the cables coming from the processor to the scope are not twisted. The processor is intended to come from the left of the patient; otherwise, the cables will drape over the patient and put undue stress on the instrument.

Intraprocedure Care of the Bronchoscope

A. Proper use of:
   1. Bite blocks: Probably the single most costly "preventable" form of damage is from not using a bite block in patients who are thought to be adequately sedated.
   2. Sedation: as above
   3. Accessories
      a. When placing accessories through the working channel, make sure that they are in the closed or "sheathed" position until they are visualized at the distal end.
      b. If at any time visualization of the accessory is lost, immediately close or resheath the accessory and retract it into the working channel to prevent damage to the patient and/or the bronchoscope.
      c. Never force an accessory through the working channel, or perforation of it can occur.
      d. When retracting an accessory from the bronchoscope, always close or resheath the accessory.
      e. If the accessory device becomes stuck in the working channel, slowly remove the bronchoscope from the patient and then attempt to remove the device, keeping the angulation in the straight position.
B. Having an extra set of eyes

As the operator has his or her eyes focused on the video monitor, it is easy to lose track of how the bronchoscope is being held or manipulated. The assistant needs to be cognizant of this and point out if the scope is being bent too acutely and suggest a correction.

Postprocedure Care of the Bronchoscope [10]

A. Initial cleaning at bedside:
   1. Wipe down insertion tube with wet gauze
   2. Flush water through scope with only the very tip submerged
   3. Suction air through for at least 10 seconds
B. Transport to cleaning area in a leakproof container that is supported on the bottom (i.e., transport tray).
C. Leak testing
   1. Apply leak test before submersing fully in water to prevent fluid invasion

2. Flex control lever for several seconds while under water to detect minute leaks

3. Observe for sufficient period of time

D. Proper disinfection, drying, and storage: Follow manufacturer's recommendations for scope reprocessing [11, 12].

DAMAGE TO THE BRONCHOSCOPE

Occasionally, or sometimes not occasionally, damage will occur to the bronchoscope [13]. The person responsible for overseeing the service should determine the cause of the damage. I would like to distinguish between damage that I would consider preventable in the hands of a careful operator versus damage that happens irrespective of the care that the operator takes in handling the equipment.

Preventable damage to the bronchoscope occurs when operators of the equipment or their assistants perform maneuvers that are not recommended with either the bronchoscope or its accessories. Simply stated, if one follows the manufacturer's recommendations, essentially most of this damage would not happen. Examples of this type of damage include:

■ Inadequate sedation to patient resulting in bites on the instrument

■ The improper use of accessories damaging the working channel [14]. When using devices like biopsy forceps, brushes, or needles, care should be taken to ensure that the sampling devices are not open during passage through the working channel of the instrument. This is by far the most common reason for damage to the channel of the scope and is completely preventable.

■ Improper transportation of the instrument leading to breakage.

Nonpreventable damage is caused by the normal wear and tear of the instrument. Examples of this type of damage include:

■ Leaks in the bending section without obvious trauma during a procedure

■ The degree of angulation of the bending section is "off" from stretching of cables

POSTDAMAGE CONSIDERATIONS

When damage does occur, one needs to consider how to deal with it. There are many questions that need to be addressed before deciding what to do. Here are some items to consider:

■ Type of damage (this will help indicate the cost of repair)

■ Age of scope

■ History of repairs

■ Is the scope under warranty? (It doesn't matter if it is from preventable damage.)

After you have this information, you can better make a determination as to whether or not to repair the instrument. At some point in the life of the scope, one needs to consider whether it is financially reasonable to repair it or whether it should be retired. This may be a scope whose useful life has expired a while ago, and you were hoping to just get another 6 months out of it before replacing it. If the decision is to retire the scope, there may still be some value in using it as a trade-in for a replacement.

If the decision is to repair it, there are many options to consider. Some of them may be:

■ Whom do I have repair it? Manufacturer versus third party?

■ What is the cost of the repair?

■ What is the turnaround time for the repair? You may not be able to go without having this scope for very long.

■ Are there loaner scopes available?

■ What are the service warranties for the repair?

PREVENTION OF DAMAGE TO THE BRONCHOSCOPE

The first step to take in prevention of future damage is to look historically at what types of damage have occurred in the past. Therefore, it is imperative to have a system in place that tracks the damage to the instrument with the type of procedure performed (including tracking those individuals performing the procedure). There needs to be a way to associate the scope used on a patient with the staff performing the procedure. (There are other infection control reasons to be able to track patients with the scope being used, but that does not pertain to this discussion). A simple logbook of repairs should be kept for each scope sent out for service. This will give you information so that when that scope is damaged in the future, then informed decisions can be made as to what the financial feasibility is for the repair.

When determinations have been made as to why damage has taken place, a plan should be developed to prevent future damage. This plan could be relatively simple, like protecting the scope from trauma during transportation, or could involve additional training of staff to make them aware of the idiosyncrasies of a particular accessory that tends to lead to damage [15].

REFERENCES

1. Ikeda S, Yanai N, Ishikawa S. Flexible bronchofiberscope. *Keio J Med.* 1968;17:1–16.
2. Mehta AC, Curtis PS, Scalzitti ML, Meeker DP. The high price of bronchoscopy. Maintenance and repair of the flexible fiberoptic bronchoscope. *Chest.* 1990;98:448–454.
3. Olympus BF-1T180 (Evis Bronchoscopy Systems Operation Manual) Olympus America Inc., Center Valley, PA, 2007.
4. Olympus CV-180 (Evis Bronchoscopy Systems Operation Manual). Olympus America Inc., Center Valley, PA, 2007.
5. Karl Stoz Endoscopy-America Inc. Non-Invasive Troubleshooting of Endoscopic Video Systems. Karl Storz Endoscopy-America Inc., Culver City, CA, 1999.
6. Olympus America Inc. How to Prevent Instrument Malfunctions for Gastrointestinal and Bronchial Endoscopes. Olympus America Inc., Center Valley, PA, 2004.
7. Mehta A, Siddiqi A, Walsh A. Prevention of damage and maintenance of a flexible bronchoscope. In: Beamis J, Mathur P, eds. *Interventional Pulmonology*, Vol. 2. New York: McGraw Hill; 1999;9–16.
8. Lee FYW. Care and maintenance of the flexible bronchoscope. In: Feinsilver SH, Fein AM, eds. *Textbook of Bronchoscopy*. Baltimore: Williams and Wilkins; 1995:100–108.
9. Prakash UBS. Bronchoscopy unit, expertise, equipment and personnel. In: Bollinger CT, Mathur PN, eds. *Interventional Bronchoscopy. Progress in Respiratory Research*. Vol. 30. Basel: Karger; 2000;31–43.
10. Olympus BF1T180 (Evis Bronchoscopy Systems Reprocessing Manual). Olympus America Inc., Center Valley, PA, 2007.
11. Culver D, Minai O, Gordon S, Mehta A. Infection control and radiation safety in the bronchoscopy suite. In: Wang K, Mehta A, Turner J, eds. *Flexible Bronchoscopy. 2nd ed.* Malden, MA : Blackwell Publishing; 2004;3:9–25.
12. Mehta A, Prakash U, Garland R, et al. American College of Chest Physicians and American Association for Bronchology Consensus Statement. Prevention of flexible bronchoscopy-associated infection. *Chest.* 2005;128:1742–1755.
13. Kirkpatrick MB, Smith JR, Hoffman PJ. Bronchoscope damage and repair costs: results of a regional postal survey. *Respir Care.* 1992;37:1256–1259.
14. Stelck M, Kulas M, Mehta A. Maintenance of the bronchoscope and bronchoscopy equipment. In: Prakash U, ed. *Bronchoscopy*. New York: Raven Press; 1994;28:381–391.
15. Lunn W, Garland R, Gryniuk L, Smith L, Feller-Kopman D, Ernst A. Reducing maintenance and repair costs in an interventional pulmonology program. *Chest.* 2005;127:1382–1387.

7

STARTING AND MANAGING A BRONCHOSCOPY UNIT

Rabih Bechara

INTRODUCTION

Pulmonary endoscopy has evolved tremendously in the past decade. Thanks to new technology, the trained pulmonologist can now perform a large array of diagnostic and therapeutic interventions. The complexity of these procedures demands training, however, and standards should be met before performing them. In addition, it is clear that the success in these procedures depends only partly on the skills of the physician; the skills of the support staff and the adequacy of the facilities and related resources are also indispensable. Increasingly, agencies such as, for example, Departments of Public Health have released regulations affecting work and workflow in endoscopy units in general.

Although pulmonologists are frequently in charge of bronchoscopy units, they are generally not prepared during a fellowship to manage these units. In fact, starting or directing a bronchoscopy unit requires substantial knowledge of the necessary staff, equipment, training, procedure space, and applicable regulations and legislation. To help provide this knowledge, I briefly describe these requirements here and comment on their importance in ensuring the success of bronchoscopic services.

THE INTAKE AND RECOVERY AREA

A dedicated intake and recovery area should be available where nurses can receive and prepare patients for procedures and to help them recover after procedures (Figures 7.1 and 7.2). Here, patients will have their medical records updated and their medications checked to be sure the procedure can be performed safely. Each patient should have his or her own space in the intake and recovery area, with curtains to provide privacy. Patients can change into the appropriate attire for the procedure, receive an identifying wrist band, have an intravenous line established, and have a place to store, for example, any loose dental appliances that must be removed before the procedure.

Each patient space should be equipped to monitor vital signs and oxygen saturation and should be sufficient to allow patients to be placed on the bed or stretcher appropriate for their procedure (that is, fluoroscopy, electromagnetic navigation, and so on).

The intake and recovery area should have at least one negative-pressure isolation room for patients who require such management. Importantly, the patient's name, attending physician, and procedures to be performed should

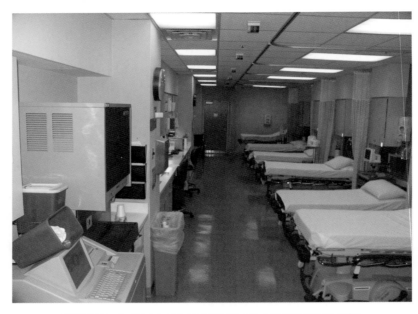

FIGURE 7.1. An intake and recovery area in a bronchoscopy suite.

be clearly displayed, and the status of the patient and the procedure should be monitored at all times, either electronically or on a schedule board, respecting patient privacy regulations.

Transportation to and from the intake and recovery area, especially to the procedure room, should be direct and without interruption; hallways should be free from clutter and competing foot traffic (Figure 7.3).

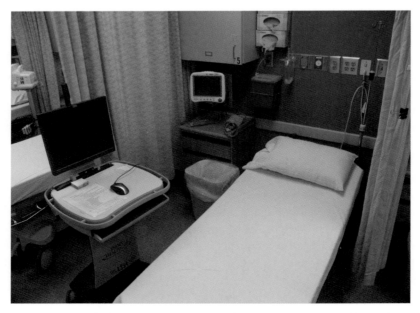

FIGURE 7.2. An individual patient space in an intake and recovery area showing monitors and a mobile workstation. Curtains secure privacy.

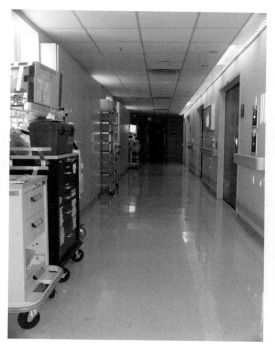

FIGURE 7.3. Hallways from the intake and recovery area to procedure rooms should always be kept clear.

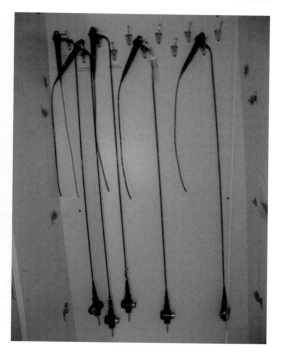

FIGURE 7.4. Bronchoscopes can be stored in the procedure room or in a nearby central location.

THE BRONCHOSCOPY PROCEDURE ROOM

Procedure rooms should be large enough to contain the equipment and staff needed to perform a specific procedure. As a rule, such rooms range between 300 and 800 square feet, but rooms dedicated to certain procedures may require more space than others. In all cases, there must be space for two individuals to stand at the head of the patient's bed, and the patient must be accessible from all sides at all times. Lighting must be sufficient and easily dimmed to maximize viewing quality during procedures. Because the electrical connections on bronchoscopes are on the left side, the processors and other equipment are usually positioned on the left side of the patient's bed, to allow easy access and to decrease potential clutter at the work site during the procedure.

Bronchoscopes can be stored in the room or in a nearby central location (Figure 7.4). After use, they should be routed immediately to a disinfection/sterilization room, which ideally is part of the suite.

Procedure rooms should also have enough space to store the equipment needed during procedures, such as tubes, slides, special media, stents, balloons, chest tubes, and so on. The locations of each item should be clearly labeled for ease of retrieval. Medications, especially for sedation, should be easily available.

Viewing monitors should be accessible to both the bronchoscopist and the assistant. If possible, monitors should be adjustable, to allow maximum flexibility in direction, height, and rotation. The number of monitors per patient varies among different centers, but each room should have at least two (Figure 7.5). Oxygen outlets, suction devices, sinks, and hand hygiene supplies should also be available in each room. In general, procedure rooms should be ventilated with negative-pressure air exchanges, and fluoroscopy rooms (for C-arm or biplanar machines) need to be able to store protective coverings for the staff (Figure 7.6).

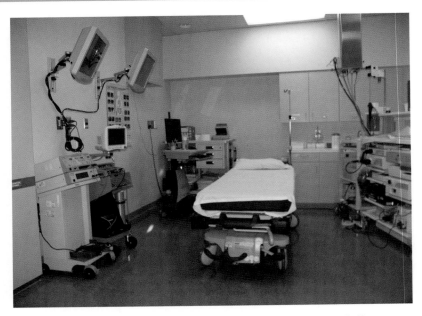

FIGURE 7.5. A basic bronchoscopy suite showing a processor (*left*).

In rooms where specimens are prepared, the work area should be free of clutter and be equipped to allow specimens to be processed promptly during the procedure. In some facilities, advanced surgical procedures are performed in bronchoscopy rooms; therefore, they need adequate overhead surgical lighting and sterile equipment (Figure 7.7). Measures to maintain the sterility of the surgical field should also be easily implemented. In such rooms, space for general

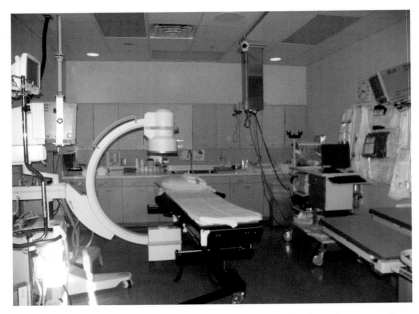

FIGURE 7.6. A C-arm fluoroscope with an appropriate bed in a bronchoscopy suite.

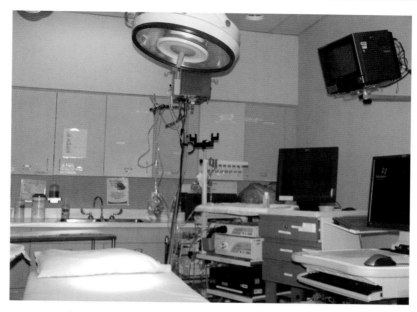

FIGURE 7.7. In some facilities, advanced surgical procedures are performed in bronchoscopy rooms, which therefore need adequate overhead surgical lighting and sterile equipment.

anaesthesia equipment must also be available. All procedure rooms should have easy access to resuscitation equipment, including airway boxes for endotracheal intubations. Cardiac defibrillators should be located in each room or in a nearby central location.

The experience that a patient has from a procedure is largely dictated by external factors, rather than the endoscopic intervention. Proper sedation, a generally pleasant atmosphere, and minimized chatter and loud noises during procedures are signs of a good endoscopy unit.

WORKSTATIONS

Proper documentation, by dictation and image, is important both for patient management and communication and for accurate billing. Thus, endoscopy suites should have dedicated workstations separate from the procedure rooms. These stations should include computers, special forms, dictation equipment, monitors, printers, and so on, and are important for completing

procedure-related paperwork. Patient-related endoscopic information should be easily available at each workstation.

ENDOSCOPY ASSISTANTS

Endoscopy assistants have important duties before, during, and after every procedure. In fact, they are very important persons in the suite: The success of the procedures depends greatly on their training, skill, and dedication. They are responsible for preparing the room, the equipment, and patients for each procedure and for handling the specimens and used equipment after the procedure.

BRONCHOSCOPY EQUIPMENT

Bronchoscopy requires a variety of equipment for performing specific diagnostic and therapeutic interventions. Equipment acquisition should thus be determined by the kind, extent, and complexity of the procedures to be undertaken in the unit. Diagnostic airway procedures and, occasionally, minimally invasive pleural procedures are common, and require the resources described below.

Several manufacturers make several different kinds of flexible bronchoscopes. Generally, all these scopes are adequate for examining the tracheobronchial tree. They range in size from ultrathin and pediatric scopes, to those with diameters of 5.3 mm and working channels of 2.0 mm for adults, to therapeutic scopes with working channels of 3.2 mm.

In units where gastrointestinal endoscopies are also performed, gastrointestinal endoscopes must be separated from bronchoscopes at all times, especially during processing, cleaning, and storage. In addition, labeling each scope and keeping accurate records of each are essential.

FLUOROSCOPY

Fluoroscopy is often useful in performing bronchoscopic procedures, including transbronchial biopsies, electromagnetic navigation, and a variety of routine pleural interventions. Radiation exposure from the recently introduced digital pulse fluoroscope is substantially lower than that from traditional fluoroscopes. When choosing a fluoroscopic system, remember that biplanar systems are more accurate than single-planar systems. Computed tomographic fluoroscopy is also available. In any case, all personnel in the fluoroscopy suite must wear dosimetry badges, and in many institutions, nonradiologists must pass a basic examination on fluoroscopic safety.

THERAPEUTIC ENDOSCOPY EQUIPMENTS

Therapeutic endoscopy equipment includes, but is not limited to, cryoprobes, cryoballoons, lasers, electrocautery, argon plasma coagulation, and airway stents. This equipment should be available in suites where therapeutic techniques, such as those for managing patients with obstructed airways, with hemoptysis secondary to endobronchial lesions, and candidates for photodynamic therapy, are performed. These patients are usually high risk; therefore, staff education and preparation should be appropriate to ensure success. In addition, comprehensive support from thoracic surgery is mandatory, especially for managing complications requiring surgery.

THE DIAGNOSIS AND MANAGEMENT OF PLEURAL DISEASE

In recent years, pulmonologists have become more involved in diagnosing and managing patients with pleural effusions, from both malignant and nonmalignant causes. Some minimally invasive pleural procedures and, more recently, invasive pleural procedures are being performed in bronchoscopy units. Thoracic ultrasonography has recently emerged as standard in imaging pleural effusions because the risk of complications during thoracocentesis is greatly reduced. Fortunately, these systems are portable and can be used in other areas as well as in bronchoscopy units.

Pleuroscopes are now available for performing invasive pleural interventions. These semirigid scopes allow visual examination and biopsy of the pleural space, and the light sources and processors are the same as those used for bronchoscopes.

SUMMARY

In summary, planning a bronchoscopy unit depends on the kinds of diagnostic and therapeutic procedures to be performed. The procedures dictate the equipment, personnel, and training necessary to perform them. Given the high risk of some patients, a comprehensive and collegial relationship with thoracic surgery is essential. The importance of staff training and preparation in the safety and success of the bronchoscopy unit cannot be overstated.

SUGGESTED READINGS

Bandoh S, Fujita J, Tojo Y, et al. Diagnostic accuracy and safety of flexible bronchoscopy with multiplanar reconstruction images and ultrafast Papanicolaou stain: evaluating solitary pulmonary nodules. *Chest.* 2003;124(5):1985–1992.

Beamis JF Jr. Interventional pulmonology techniques for treating malignant large airway obstruction: an update. *Curr Opin Pulmon Med.* 2005;11(4):292–295.

Haas AR, Sterman DH, Musani AI. Malignant pleural effusions: management options with consideration of coding, billing, and a decision approach. *Chest.* 2007;132(3):1036–1041.

Herth FJ. Eberhardt R, Ernst A. The future of bronchoscopy in diagnosing, staging and treatment of lung cancer. *Respiration.* 2006;73(4):399–409.

Jain P, Pleming P, Mehta A. Radiation safety for healthcare workers in the bronchoscopy suite. *Clin Chest Med.* 1999;20(1):33–38, ix–x.

Mathur PN, Loddenkemper R. Medical thoracoscopy. Role in pleural and lung diseases. *Clin Chest Med.* 1995;16(3):487–496.

Shulman L, Ost D. Advances in bronchoscopic diagnosis of lung cancer. *Curr Opin Pulmon Med.* 2007;13(4):271–277.

8

FLEXIBLE BRONCHOSCOPY: INDICATIONS, CONTRAINDICATIONS, AND CONSENT

Aaron B. Waxman

INTRODUCTION

The ability of the bronchoscope to provide either diagnostic data or a therapeutic intervention is changing with technology. Improvements in digital imaging and materials along with newer interfaces utilizing positioning technology and diagnostic imaging are enhancing the capabilities of flexible bronchoscopy. Thus the role of flexible bronchoscopy in practice is changing and will depend on the facilities available at a particular center. This review will go over the broad indications and the relatively few contraindications for flexible bronchoscopy based on the current state of the art. The considerations important for obtaining informed consent as it pertains to flexible bronchoscopy will also be reviewed.

INDICATIONS FOR FLEXIBLE BRONCHOSCOPY

Indications for flexible bronchoscopy are often thought of in terms of diagnosis and therapy. For diagnostic bronchoscopy, we can divide areas broadly into endobronchial signs and symptoms, findings from diagnostic studies such as chest radiography, and those based on specific injuries that may impact the airways. Symptoms and signs of endobronchial disease are the most common indications for flexible bronchoscopy and

include chronic cough, hemoptysis, focal unexplained atelectasis, or a postobstructive pneumonia. Findings on examination can also be indications for flexible bronchoscopy including a localized wheeze, which could be the result of something partially blocking an airway. Patients with what sounds like refractory "asthma" or focal findings of wheezing on examination, or altered breath sounds associated with a radiographic finding may be appropriate indications (Figure 8.1). Patients who have abnormal flow volume curves may have obstructing lesions in the large airways that can easily be assessed by use of a flexible bronchoscope. Although stridor may be considered a tempting indication for taking a look, any patient with stridor needs to be approached with great caution and with a well-planned approach to the difficult airway. Findings that can cause changes in examination of the chest or respiratory symptoms might include an endobronchial neoplasm, broncholithiasis, stricture or stenosis of large airways, foreign body aspiration, extrinsic compression of an airway by a parenchymal or mediastinal tumor or lymph node, a bronchopleural fistula, paradoxical vocal cord dysfunction, or the carcinoid syndrome. Very often an abnormal chest radiograph will result in a referral for flexible bronchoscopy. Findings that raise concern and are indications for flexible bronchoscopy include an obvious mass lesion or a recurring pulmonary infiltrate in the same anatomical region that

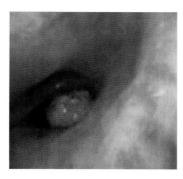

FIGURE 8.1. Broncholith in a patient with a persistent focal wheeze on physical examination despite maximal therapy for asthma.

may signal an obstructive lesion (Figure 8.2). Persistent atelectasis could signal a compressive lesion or endobronchial obstruction caused by a tumor or foreign body. Mediastinal abnormalities such as enlarged lymph nodes that are abutting the trachea and accessible by transtracheal or transbronchial needle biopsy may be seen on chest radiograph or computed tomography of the chest. Likewise, diffuse parenchymal disease such as sarcoidosis may be approached with the bronchoscope for a diagnosis (Figure 8.3). In other cases of interstitial lung disease, flexible bronchoscopic sampling may not provide enough tissue

for a definitive diagnosis, and thoracoscopic or open lung biopsy may still be required.

One of the most important indications for bronchoscopy is in the diagnosis of lung cancer. The bronchoscope can be used for making a tissue diagnosis via endobronchial, transbronchial, or needle biopsy; for staging of lung cancer with transtracheal lymph node biopsy; or for early diagnosis in the setting of chronic cough or abnormal chest radiograph in the appropriate patient [1,2].

Patients who suffer traumatic injuries may require bronchoscopy to assess the extent of injury. This might include patients who have suffered extensive burn or thermal injury and are suspected of having injuries to the lower airways. Because these patients may have significant debris or tissue damage, diagnostic bronchoscopy may be combined with therapeutic bronchoscopy for purposes of rinsing out debris or necrotic tissue. Likewise, patients who have suffered blunt or penetrating thoracic trauma may require bronchoscopy to assess for bronchial disruption or fracture. Finally, in the intensive care unit in patients who are intubated, bronchoscopy can be used for assessment of endotracheal tube position.

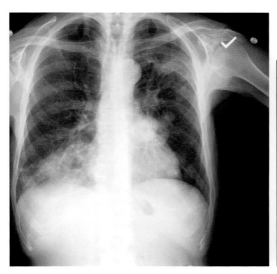

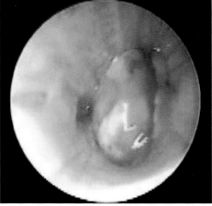

FIGURE 8.2. Chest radiograph (*left*) from patient with recurrent pneumonia. Bronchoscopy (*right*) revealed an obstructive lesion in the right lower lobe.

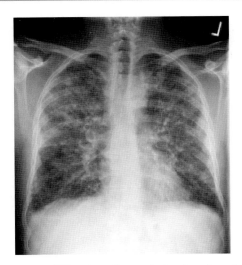

FIGURE 8.3. Diffuse lung disease that on transbronchial biopsy was consistent with sarcoidosis.

Therapeutic bronchoscopy covers a number of areas. One of the more important and often difficult indications for flexible bronchoscopy is in the removal of a foreign body. In general, foreign body removal is best done with a rigid bronchoscope under general anesthesia. Flexible bronchoscopy can be used as an initial screening procedure for suspected cases of aspiration. Patients with known or suspected foreign bodies should undergo rigid bronchoscopy. If the evidence for aspiration is equivocal, patients should undergo diagnostic flexible bronchoscopy. If a foreign body is found, a rigid bronchoscopy can follow. In certain rare cases, a foreign body extraction can be done with a flexible bronchoscope.

When a patient presents with lung abscess, flexible bronchoscopy can be performed to rule out endobronchial obstruction as a result of a foreign body or a mass lesion. In certain cases, the bronchoscope can be used for drainage of the abscess cavity. Other indications may include tracheal stenosis requiring dilation and possible stenting, or refractory atelectasis [3] that may benefit from a balloon dilatation.

Occasionally, flexible bronchoscopy will be indicated for respiratory toilet. As a general rule, postural drainage, cough, and suction of secretions are sufficient. If for some reason these cannot be done, then bronchoscopy can be used for respiratory toilette. Prospective studies have shown that intensive respiratory toilette can accomplish good results in the control of atelectasis [for review, see 4]. However, there are many clinical circumstances in which respiratory toilette cannot ideally be accomplished. These include immobilized patients, patients with spine or spinal cord injury, patients with thoracic trauma such as flail chest, postoperative patients in whom pain is a significant issue, or patients supported with an aortic balloon pump. Some bronchoscopists advocate treating left lower lobe atelectasis with the flexible bronchoscope and lavage. In general, blind passage of a mini-bronchoalveolar lavage (BAL) catheter or blind suctioning in the intubated patient with in-line catheters is difficult to direct to specific regions such as the left lower lobe. In cases in which it is important to verify where a sample is obtained, flexible bronchoscopy provides obvious benefit.

Flexible bronchoscopy may serve as a prelude to other procedures or interventions. In patients with pneumonia or diffuse lung disease, bronchoscopy can be performed to obtain respiratory secretions for establishing the diagnosis of an infection. The choice of brushing, protected brush specimen, or BAL is dependent on the clinical situation and can be done following airway inspection.

If difficulty is experienced in performing an intubation, or if a difficult intubation is anticipated, a flexible bronchoscope can be used. The endotracheal tube is placed over the flexible bronchoscope. After the bronchoscope is advanced through the vocal cords and is in a good position, the endotracheal tube is passed over the bronchoscope and, under direct vision, can be introduced into the trachea and its position verified.

There are a number of conditions in which flexible bronchoscopy may not be helpful. This is dependent on the state of available technology and the experience of the bronchoscopist. An important example is the peripheral solitary pulmonary nodule beyond the reach of the

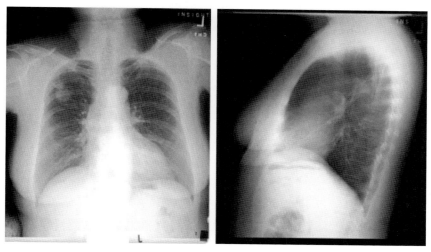

FIGURE 8.4. Peripheral right upper lobe lesion that may not be readily accessible by conventional flexible bronchoscopy.

bronchoscope (Figure 8.4). Furthermore, there is no role for bronchoscopy in the setting of an isolated pleural effusion or a chronic cough in a patient who is younger than 55, with a clear chest radiograph, and no smoking history or risk factors for lung cancer. Acute stridor in children is a medical emergency and an absolute contraindication for bronchoscopy. In cases of uncomplicated pneumonia, either community- or hospital-acquired pneumonia, bronchoscopy often adds little information and has no impact on medical decision making. Last, in cases of massive hemoptysis, the flexible bronchoscope is often too small and ineffective in clearing blood fast enough to prevent occlusion of the airway or to find and treat a source of bleeding. Rigid bronchoscopy is the preferred approach to massive hemoptysis.

CONTRAINDICATIONS TO FLEXIBLE BRONCHOSCOPY

To date there have not been any trials to assess those factors that may increase the risk for patients undergoing flexible bronchoscopy. The decision to perform flexible bronchoscopy, like that for any procedure, must be made after weighing the potential benefits of the procedure against the potential risk to the patient. In general, most contraindications to flexible bronchoscopy are relative rather than absolute and are based on common sense. There should be available to the bronchoscopist adequate facilities and personnel to handle emergencies that could occur during the procedure, including cardiopulmonary arrest, pneumothorax, or bleeding. An inability to adequately oxygenate the patient during the procedure based on his or her clinical presentation is a clear contraindication to performing bronchoscopy, particularly in a nonintubated patient. When assessing a patient before the procedure, special attention must be paid to his or her respiratory status and potential for clinical decline as a result of the procedure, including patients with severe obstructive airway disease, patients with severe refractory hypoxemia, or patients with an unstable hemodynamic status. Likewise, assessment of a patient's bleeding status is critical, especially when biopsies are being considered. The procedure may need to be postponed for a patient whose coagulopathy or bleeding diathesis cannot be corrected.

Relative contraindications to this, or any procedure, might include lack of patient cooperation, a recent myocardial infarction or unstable angina, a partial tracheal obstruction, moderate-to-severe hypoxemia, or hypercarbia. Depending on available facilities and comorbidities, additional relative contraindications might include morbid obesity or severe sleep apnea. It is preferable that patients do not undergo elective conscious sedation until 8 hours after a solid meal or 2–4 hours after clear liquids or medications given orally.

HAZARDS AND COMPLICATIONS OF FLEXIBLE BRONCHOSCOPY

Even though flexible bronchoscopy is a relatively safe and well-tolerated procedure, there are still a number of potential complications, which can include airway problems (including those that result from irritation including laryngospasm, increased airway resistance, exacerbation of obstructive airways disease, and physical obstruction). There can be mechanical problems including epistaxis, hemoptysis, or pneumothorax. Complications can be directly hemodynamically important such as cardiac arrhythmias, including bradycardia, or other vagally mediated phenomena, tachyarrhythmias, or cardiac arrest. The bronchoscopes themselves can pose a hazard to both the bronchoscopist and the patient through exposure to infection. Cross-contamination of specimens or bronchoscopes has also occurred. In general, flexible bronchoscopy is usually an extraordinarily safe procedure with major complications, such as bleeding, respiratory depression, and pneumothorax, occurring in less than 1% of cases [5,6] Mortality is rare, with a reported death rate of 0%–0.04% in a large number of procedures [5,6].

CONSENT AND PRESCREENING

When obtaining consent, start out with a clear explanation of the procedure. Using a finger, show the size of the bronchoscope, or show the patient the actual bronchoscope, to allay his or her anxieties. Everyone fears suffocation and

gagging, so it is important to assure the patient that there is sufficient room for air to go through the throat while the scope is in the airway. Explain how the gag reflex and gagging are alleviated, in most cases, with topical lidocaine. This will also help to decrease coughing. Make it clear to the patient that the scope is going to pass through the vocal cords and that he or she should try not to talk during the procedure as it can cause damage to the vocal cords. Recall that there is no pain sensation within the lung; only the pleura are innervated with pain fibers, so the patient should not feel any pain during a flexible bronchoscopy. The response to irritation in the lung is to cough, and coughing is suppressed with topical anesthetics. Work out hand signals so that the patient can let you know how he or she is doing or can answer any questions without talking.

Prior to the procedure, a preprocedure screen is completed that includes obtaining a history of allergic reactions to local anesthetic. If clinically indicated, blood urea nitrogen (>30 mg/dL), creatinine (>3.0 mg/dL), platelet count ($<50,000$), prothrombin time, and partial thromboplastin time will be checked, especially if biopsies are being considered. If indicated, a complete blood count should also be checked. In appropriate circumstances we will evaluate for evidence of a recent myocardial infarction or active cardiac issues. There should be an evaluation of American Society of Anesthesiologists (ASA) class and a proper airway assessment such as the Mallampati grade or equivalent. In many centers, patients graded as an ASA III or higher are required to have an electrocardiogram within the past 6 months or if there are risk factors for myocardial disease. Everyone is encouraged to review their center-specific protocols before administering conscious sedation.

INFORMED CONSENT

Informed consent is obtained for all therapeutic and diagnostic procedures. In all cases, the patient (or a patient's surrogate) should give consent voluntarily. Regardless of who is giving

MASSACHUSETTS GENERAL HOSPITAL

PATIENT IDENTIFICATION AREA

PROCEDURE CONSENT FORM

PATIENT:

UNIT NO:

PROCEDURE:

☐ Right   ☐ Left   ☐ Bilateral   ☐ Not applicable

Patient's Name!

I have explained to the patient/family/guardian the nature of the patient's condition, the nature of the procedure, and the benefits to be reasonably expected compared with alternative approaches. I have discussed the likelihood of major risks or complications of this procedure including (if applicable) but not limited to drug reactions, hemorrhage, infection, complications from blood or blood components. I have also indicated that with any procedure there is always the possibility of an unexpected complication.

☐ I have given the patient written teaching materials to help inform him/her.

☒ Conscious sedation is being used for this procedure and I have explained that risks include suppressed breathing, low blood pressure and occasionally incomplete pain relief.

☒ The following additional issues were discussed.

- **Low Blood Oxygen**
- **Difficulty breathing that might require oxygen, assisted breathing, or admission to the intensive care unit**
- **Adverse Drug Reaction**
- **Abnormal Heart Rhythm**
- **Fever**
- **Infection**
- **Sore Throat**
- **Air Leak Around The Lung With Lung Collapse**
- **Death**

☒ All questions were answered and the patient/family/guardian consents to the procedure.

_____
(Physician/Licensed Practitioner that is performing the procedure (Signature)

DATE: **Today's Date!** _____

Time: _____ AM / PM

Dr. Waxman
_____   has explained the above to me and I consent to the procedure.

I understand that Massachusetts General Hospital is an academic medical center and that residents, fellows and students in medical and allied disciplines may participate in this procedure. At times observers may be present, as considered appropriate or advisable by the surgeon/attending or his/her associate and in accordance with hospital policy. Since aspects of this procedure may have educational or scientific value, data, video or photographs may be obtained for teaching purposes, presentations at medical/scientific meetings or publications in a medical/scientific journals. In addition, I understand that blood or other specimens removed for necessary diagnostic or therapeutic reasons may later be disposed of by MGH. These materials also may be used by MGH, its affiliates, or other academic or commercial entities, for research, educational purposes (including photography), or other activity, if it furthers the Hospital's missions.

Patient's Signature!
_____
(patient's/health care agent's/guardian's/family's signature*)

*(If patient's signature cannot be obtained, indicate reason in comments section above.)

10465 (12/06)

FIGURE 8.5. Example of a consent form used for flexible bronchoscopy.

consent (the patient or his or her proxy), you should be certain that he or she is competent to provide consent. It is good practice that the information about the procedure is provided by a person who is participating in the procedure. Consent should be worded in plain English (or with the assistance of an appropriate interpreter) at no more than an eighth grade reading and comprehension level. In every case you should clearly explain the rationale, the inherent risks, the potential benefits for the procedure, and any alternatives to the procedure (Table 8.1 and

Table 8.1. *Suggested wording of potential complications while explaining the risks of flexible bronchoscopy to a patient*

- Low blood oxygen
- Difficulty breathing that might require oxygen, assisted breathing, or admission to the intensive care unit
- Adverse drug reaction
- Abnormal heart rhythm
- Fever
- Infection
- Sore throat
- Air leak around the lung with lung collapse
- Death

Figure 8.5). Consent should be obtained prior to any sedation being given to the patient. After the patient is under sedation, he or she may misinterpret or forget what you say. When discussing the procedure with the patient, make it clear to him or her that results should not be expected right away. Microbiologic results can take days to weeks. Cytology and pathology evaluation can take several days for tissue processing and evaluation before results are available.

REFERENCES

1. Mazzone P, Jain P, Arroliga AC, Matthay RA. Bronchoscopy and needle biopsy techniques for diagnosis and staging of lung cancer. *Clin Chest Med.* 2002;23(1):137–158, ix.
2. Herth FJ, Eberhardt R, Ernst A. The future of bronchoscopy in diagnosing, staging and treatment of lung cancer. *Respiration.* 2006;73(4):399–409.
3. Kreider ME, Lipson DA. Bronchoscopy for atelectasis in the ICU: a case report and review of the literature. *Chest.* 2003;124(1):344–350.
4. Pryor JA. Physiotherapy for airway clearance in adults. *Eur Respir J.* 1999;14(6):1418–1424.
5. de Blic J, Marchac V, Scheinmann P. Complications of flexible bronchoscopy in children: prospective study of 1,328 procedures. *Eur Respir J.* 2002;20(5):1271–1276.
6. Borchers SD, Beamis JF Jr. Flexible bronchoscopy. *Chest Surg Clin North Am.* 1996;6(2):169–192.

9

BRONCHIAL WASHING, BRONCHOALVEOLAR LAVAGE, BRONCHIAL BRUSH, AND ENDOBRONCHIAL BIOPSY

Carla Lamb

There is often a complementary role of bronchial washing (BW) or bronchoalveolar lavage (BAL), bronchial brushing, and endobronchial biopsy (EBBX). One or more of them is performed with transbronchial needle aspirate and transbronchial lung biopsy. This review is to provide the bronchoscopist a practical guide to procedural decision making in terms of specimen collection and diagnostic approach. Each of these procedures will be defined and techniques discussed. The role they play in diagnosis alone or in combination in infectious disease, drug-induced lung disease, inflammatory and occupational lung disease, and in malignant diseases is explained. General indications for these procedures, identification of key elements of specimen collection methods, diagnostic information that can be obtained, and advances in technology is reviewed.

When approaching the patient with an abnormal chest radiograph or computed tomography (CT) scan, it is important to plan a strategy of questions to be answered and specimens to be collected well before the bronchoscopic procedure even begins. It is worthwhile to create a broad differential diagnosis based on the patient history specifically in terms of immunocompetence, medication and environmental exposures, infectious contacts, and travel. Risk factors for malignancy should be assessed. Chest imaging will identify extent and location of disease. These variables will determine the bronchoscopic tests

to be ordered and the location of the sample to be obtained as well as the quantity of specimen required. Communication with the bronchoscopy team is essential to ensure the preparation of the proper tools for specimen retrieval and collection, as well as appropriate respiratory isolation of the patient and staff in specific clinical settings. Communication with the microbiology and the cytology departments is also important. Listing a patient's specific differential diagnosis when completing the cytology lab request forms will improve the cytopathologic review by alerting the pathologist to your clinical concerns. The general indications and contraindications for bronchoscopy are discussed in another chapter. Specific individual procedural risks will be cited where relevant in this chapter.

BRONCHIAL WASHING

Collection of BWs most often occurs in the simultaneous setting of bronchial brushings and biopsies for cytology. When reviewing its yield relative to these, some describe that BW offers little over the combination brush and biopsy. It should be distinguished from the more standardized BAL. BWs do not require wedging the bronchoscope into a subsegmental position, and the volume of saline flushed into the desired bronchial site is far less, ranging from 5 to 50 mL. It is often used as a means for assisting bronchial pulmonary toilet by dislodging a mucus plug or clot. The lower volumes of instilled saline required may be desirable in the more marginal patient in whom BAL would be intolerable. Although it can be used to diagnose infection, true bacterial quantification for diagnosing pneumonia is limited because of both specimen size and the high potential for respiratory flora contamination. Generally 5–15 mL of fluid will be required for basic microbiologic evaluation, and 10 mL for cytology. It is also felt that washings should be performed prior to biopsies to avoid excess red blood cells that sometimes obscure cytologic interpretation, although it has been described that the sequence of the wash before or after biopsy in the presence of an endobronchial lesion did not impact diagnostic yield and resulted in 57% and 55% in prebiopsy and postbiopsy washes, respectively. BW did appear to increase overall diagnostic yield when performed in conjunction with biopsy in endobronchial tumor to 96% compared with biopsy alone at 93%. Acute infection may create atypical squamous metaplasia that can be nearly impossible to differentiate from malignancy and must be interpreted with caution in the appropriate clinical context. Generally, limiting the use of topical lidocaine to less than 3 mL prior to specimen collection will reduce any bactericidal effect on the diagnostic yield in microbiology specimens. BAL is considered superior to BW in all aspects of analysis primarily because of its volume and avoidance of large airway respiratory cell contamination.

BRONCHOALVEOLAR LAVAGE

BAL, although not universally standardized, has evolved as a minimally invasive means to assist in specific diagnosis across the spectrum of benign and malignant pulmonary diseases, to measure exacerbations of certain diseases, and to evaluate response to therapy. Research protocols over the past three to four decades have played a significant part in establishing a more defined role of the BAL technique as part of routine flexible bronchoscopy. As a form of liquid lung biopsy, it is felt to represent millions of alveoli as well as the respiratory epithelial lining. Knowledge of the range of cellular findings in normal individuals is necessary to assess adequacy of sampling as well as to define pathologic findings. Cellular contents in BAL of normal controls consist of 95% macrophages, 3% lymphocytes, and 1%–2% neutrophils, eosinophils, or basophils. Paucity of excessive epithelial cells and erythrocytes is desired. An unsatisfactory sample may be defined as the lack of alveolar macrophages, excessive airway epithelial cells ($>5\%$), and an abundance of purulent material from the central airways. Lavage plays its most significant role in identifying infection in both immunocompromised and immunocompetent patients, identifying malignancy, and assessing cellular components in study protocols that mark disease activity in asthma and interstitial lung diseases.

A common approach to BAL collection following bronchoscopic airway inspection is as a unilateral lung lavage obtained in the most abnormal lung and sampled in at least two subsegmental regions or right middle lobe or lingula in diffuse disease. It is notable that the latter two segments render the best volume yield. The isotonic, nonbacteriostatic sterile saline used may be warmed or kept at room temperature with a total volume of 100–300 mL instilled sequentially as 20- to 50-mL aliquots up to 4 to 5 times. Each aliquot can be aspirated manually with a 20-mL syringe through the bronchoscopic working channel or by use of a sterile collection trap connected to suction while partially depressing the bronchoscopic suction channel to avoid airway trauma from collapse of the bronchi around the bronchoscope. Delaying immediate retrieval of the instilled saline over a few seconds and allowing the patient to breathe two or so respiratory cycles may provide better mixing. Many clinicians will remove the first aspirated return and discard this as it represents the proximal bronchial contents. The patient's spontaneous movement or coughing may dislodge the bronchoscope and disrupt the wedge position. The wedge position should be at the level of the third- to fourth-order bronchi (Figure 9.1). There is a balance of maintaining the snug wedge position to ensure that the saline instilled does not escape around the bronchoscope while not advancing the bronchoscope too far in order to avoid inducing trauma to the bronchial mucosa and may result in contamination and overall poor sampling of the distal alveoli during specimen collection. BAL should be performed prior to brush and biopsy so as not to obscure the cellular contents with trauma-induced red blood cells. Ideally, it is important to avoid suctioning while passing the nasopharynx and central airways prior to BAL, as well as to limit the amount of lidocaine (<3 mL) instilled via the working channel, as both can alter the cellular yield of the specimen. A small amount of sterile saline can be flushed through the working channel prior to specimen collection to attempt to clear it of any debris. A return volume of approximately half of the volume originally instilled is the goal.

The role of BAL is best described based on specific disease entities that deserve review and will be briefly highlighted. In general, BAL plays the most significant role in identifying infection.

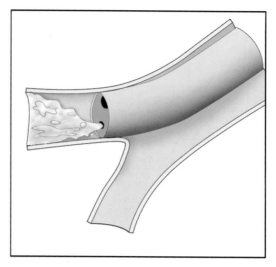

FIGURE 9.1 Wedge position of the bronchoscope for BAL in the third- to fourth-order subsegmental bronchi. (Illustration by Carla Lamb and Vinald Francis.)

The bronchoscopist should be aware of the studies that can be sent on a BAL sample (Table 9.1). In some disease entities, BAL may be used as a stand-alone test for diagnosis in a number of infectious and inflammatory lung diseases. Although the presence of certain findings is definitive for pathogenesis, other findings may not correlate directly with actual disease, and

Table 9.1. *Studies for BW, BAL, bronchial brush, and EBBX*

BW/BAL	Brush	EBBX
AFB/modified AFB (Kinyoun)	AFB	AFB
Fungal stains/culture	Fungal	Fungal
Bacterial (quantitative)	Bacterial Clt (Quant)	Bacterial Clt
Viral	Viral	Viral
Legionella (DFA/Clt)		
Silver stain for *Pneumocystis*		
PCR for tuberculosis		
PCR for *Pneumocystis*		
Galactomannan for *Aspergillus*		
Cell count and differential		
CD4-to-CD8 ratio		
Cytology	Cytology	Cytopathology
Flow cytometry (cell markers)		Flow cytometry (for lymphoma)

Note: AFB, acid-fast bacilli; Clt, culture; DFA, direct fluorescence antibody; PCR, polymerase chain reaction.

Table 9.2. *Role of BAL in infectious disease states*

If Identified in BAL	
Pathogenic	**Use clinical context** **May not be pathogenic**
• Bacteria predominant 10,000 cfu/mL • *Histoplasma capsulatum*, Blastomycetes, Coccidioidomycosis • Influenza • *Legionella*	• *Aspergillus* • Atypical *Mycobacterium* • *Candida* • *Cryptococcus*
• *Mycobacterium* tuberculosis • *Mycoplasma* • *Pneumocystis jiroveci* • Respiratory syncytial virus • *Strongyloides* (other parasitic organisms) • *Toxoplasma gondii*	• Cytomegalovirus • Herpes simplex

Adapted from: *Am J Respir Crit Care Med*. 1990;142:481–486.

their presence must be interpreted in the clinical context of the patient (Tables 9.2–9.4). BAL also has a role in diagnosis and assessment of response to therapy, but often is considered as a complementary study to additional biopsy specimens. Some general indications for BAL include diffuse alveolar or interstitial lung disease, unresolving pneumonia, alveolar hemorrhage, abnormal chest imaging in the immunocompromised host, diagnosis of ventilator-associated pneumonia (VAP) or other infections, malignancy, and research assessments for alveolar cellular content. The key is to approach the patient with a strategy of the type of analysis to be performed,

decide if BAL alone will answer the diagnostic question, review chest images to determine site of collection, adhere to a standardized technique, and confirm wedge position throughout the procedure.

In performing any bronchoscopic procedure, appropriate precautions and patient selection apply to the diagnostic procedures discussed here and are reviewed in greater detail in other chapters. Potential complications may occur with BAL and include fever (2%); pneumonitis (0.4%); pneumonia, hypoxemia, respiratory failure, or hemorrhage (0.7%); and bronchospasm (0.7%). Rarely, pneumothorax may be encountered.

Table 9.3. *Role of BAL in noninfectious diseases*

Diagnostic	Suggestive, not definitive
Pulmonary alveolar proteinosis Langerhans cell histiocytosis Lipoid pneumonia/Fat embolism Malignancy	Alveolar hemorrhage Asbestosis Berylliosis Drug-induced disease (amiodarone) Eosinophilic pneumonias Hypersensitivity pneumonitis Sarcoidosis Silicosis

Adapted from: *Am J Respir Crit Care Med*. 1990;142:481–486.

Table 9.4. *Disease associations with BAL studies/findings*

Microbiologic	Cytologic
KOH: fungal	Sulfur granules: actinomycetes
India ink: *Cryptococcus*	Hemosiderin-laden macrophages (alveolar hemorrhage) >20% red blood cells
Modified acid fast: *Nocardia*	Foamy macrophages: amiodarone, alveolar proteinosis, *Pneumocystis*
Ziehl-Neelsen, Auramine O: *Mycobacteria*	Malignancies
Silver methenamine: *Pneumocystis*/fungal	Oil Red O stain: fat embolism
Gram stain: predominant bacterial	Sudan stain: lipoid pneumonia
	>20% eosinophils: acute or chronic eosinophilic pneumonia, allergic bronchopulmonary aspergillosis, Churg–Strauss toxic inhalation, drug reaction
	Increased CD4-to-CD8 ratio: sarcoidosis, berylliosis, asbestosis, connective tissue disease
	Decreased CD4-to-CD8 ratio: hypersensitivity pneumonitis, silicosis, drug-induced disease, rheumatoid disease
	Periodic acid-Schiff: alveolar proteinosis
	Flow cytometry: lymphoma

Another unique complication is that of broncho-scopic transmission of infection. For example, outbreaks of *mycobacterium* and other bacterial infections have been a result of improper cleaning techniques, failure to perform postprocedural leak tests, and faulty bronchoscopic working channels. Prophylactic antibiotics should be considered for patients who are asplenic, have a prosthetic heart valve, or have a history of prior endocarditis (level C recommendation, British Thoracic Society guidelines). It has been found that BAL can be safely performed in the coagulopathic, immunocompromised patient. The need for diagnostic data may be significant enough to require elective intubation to secure the airway and allow for BAL sampling. This is often seen in the immunocompromised patient presenting with acute hypoxemia and radiographic evidence of diffuse airspace disease.

Specimen handling and processing from the bronchoscopy suite to the microbiology and cytology labs are as important as the methods of collection during the procedure. Ideally, specimens should be processed within 1–4 hours of collection or refrigerated if a delay is anticipated. BAL fluid should be transported on ice or at room temperature if it can be processed within the hour of collection. The exact volume of fluid required for specific tests can be slightly variable (generally, 5–10 mL of BAL fluid for Gram stain, fungal, and routine cultures; 20 mL for cell count and differential, fungal, viral, *Legionella*, *Pneumocystis*, *Nocardia*; 5–10 mL for flow cytometry/cell markers; and 15 mL for cytology). For a more detailed review of specimen processing technique, see Suggested Readings.

ROLE OF BRONCHOALVEOLAR LAVAGE IN DISEASE-SPECIFIC ENTITIES

VAP

VAP is a disease process in which BAL may have a specific role not only to assist with identification of a pathogen, but to simultaneously rule out other noninfectious etiologies for airspace disease in the intensive care patient with respiratory failure. The method of collection is as described above; however, there is also a protected BAL (pBAL) method with a balloon catheter to reduce proximal airway contamination of cultures by creating a barrier and sealing the airway orifice with the balloon while the saline is flushed through the distal catheter into the desired airway lumen. Collection of specimens prior to antibiotic initiation or within 48 hours of antibiotics is recommended. Avoiding inadvertent contact of the bronchoscope tip to the external environment of the patient is also important to avoid contamination of the instrument. VAP is defined with quantitative BAL cultures of 10,000 colony-forming units (cfu) per milliliter of a predominant pathogen (or, if there is a strong clinical suspicion, 1000–10,000 cfu/mL). Protected specimen brush (PSB) performed by bronchoscopy will be discussed later in this chapter. Other less invasive methods of diagnosing VAP are frequently compared with BAL and PSB and include nonbronchoscopic BAL, as well as blind PSB. Nonbronchoscopic BAL in a number of studies was found to be as successful as more invasive bronchoscopic methods. Bronchoscopy is performed at greater expense, requires trained personnel, and in analysis has not had an impact on patient mortality. Both bronchoscopic and nonbronchoscopic BAL have allowed for de-escalation of broad-spectrum antibiotics and offer secondary cost benefits with potential reduction of development of resistant nosocomial bacteria.

Fungal Pneumonias

The presence of *Histoplasma capsulatum*, *Blastomyces dermatitidis*, or *Coccidioides immitis* signifies pathogenesis when present in BAL. Although very often considered a pathogen, *Cryptococcus neoformans* can colonize the airway in some instances and must be interpreted in the clinical context of the individual patient. The organisms can be detected on Gram stain and silver stain along with fungal cultures.

Although the presence of *Aspergillus* may not represent pathogenicity in all cases, in the appropriate clinical context of an immuno-compromised host in the critical care setting it should be strongly considered. Assessing for invasive *Aspergillus* is necessary. The yield on BAL cytology and culture for *Aspergillus* is 40%–50%. An additional study to identify *Aspergillus* is galactomannan (GM) in BAL. This is a tool used in the intensive care setting as an early diagnostic tool for invasive aspergillosis. It is the measurement of the presence of an exoantigen released from the *Aspergillus* hyphae. It is part of the polysaccharide fungal cell wall that is released during invasion into the patient's tissues. This enzyme-linked immunosorbent assay (ELISA) has a sensitivity of GM detection of 88% and a specificity of 87%. Of note, β-lactam antibiotics can cause a false-positive result.

Mycobacterium tuberculosis

In patients unable to expectorate a sputum sample, or when induced sputum with hypertonic saline is nondiagnostic, BAL should be performed. Bronchoscopic specimens are reported as smear positive in 35%–45% of cases and in cultures in up to 90%. In miliary tuberculosis, the yield can approach 100%. BAL and BWs were found to be more sensitive than transbronchial biopsies in the HIV/AIDS population. The combined use of bronchoalveolar fluid smear and *Mycobacterium* complex polymerase chain reaction (PCR) offers a relatively good diagnostic yield in patients with smear-negative tuberculosis and in those without sputum production. It is also useful to distinguish nontuberculous *mycobacterium* from tuberculous disease.

Tropical Pneumonias

There is a wide range of pathogens and diseases that make up the tropical infectious pneumonias. Bronchoscopy with BAL may be helpful in a number of these, which include *Burkholderia pseudomallei* (melioidosis, nocardiosis, *Cryptococcus neoformans*, tuberculosis, coccidioidomycosis, paracoccidioidomycosis, *Syngamus laryngeus* (syngamosis), hookworm, paragonimiasis, amebiasis, *Echinococcus*, filariasis, *Strongyloides*, ascariasis, and toxoplasmosis.

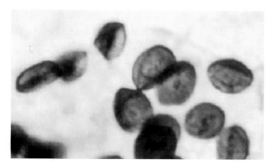

FIGURE 9.2 *Pneumocystis jiroveci* as seen in BAL specimen with silver stain.

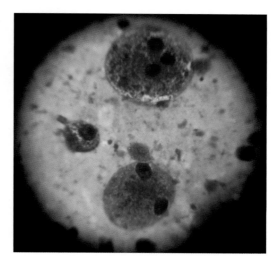

FIGURE 9.3 Alveolar macrophages filled engorged with PAS-positive material in PAP.

Immunocompromised Host

BAL in the immunocompromised host ranging from the HIV patient, to medically induced immunosuppression, to granulocytopenic patients with hematologic malignancy, to the organ transplant population, is most helpful to assess for opportunistic infections and drug-induced lung disease as a stand-alone procedure. Of note, although BAL did result in a diagnosis and resultant change of therapy based on the data, it did not impact the long-term outcome of these patients. It is complementary to brush, EBBX, and transbronchial biopsy for assessment of organ rejection in lung transplantation and secondary malignancies. In the setting of allograft rejection, the increased presence of lymphocytes along with biopsy evaluation helped diagnose these patients.

An organism that deserves special mention in the immunocompromised population is *Pneumocystis jiroveci* (Figure 9.2). BAL sensitivity exceeds 90% and is always a pathogen when this is found in bronchoalveolar fluid. It may become more difficult to identify this organism beyond 10–15 days into a treatment course. It is identified by Diff-Quik stain (Baxter Diagnostics, Inc, McGaw Park, IL) or methenamine silver stain. PCR may have a role in even earlier diagnoses. These assays have detected *Pneumocystis* DNA in BAL, biopsy, and even oropharyngeal washings obtained by mouth rinsing.

Pulmonary Alveolar Proteinosis

BAL plays a significant role in the diagnosis of pulmonary alveolar proteinosis (PAP) by the appearance of milky alveolar lavage material with sediment, cytologic analysis demonstrating the positive periodic acid-Schiff (PAS) stain of the proteinaceous material that fills the alveolar spaces, and alveolar macrophages, although few in number, are stuffed with eosinophilic granules or PAS-positive material (Figure 9.3). The macrophages become overwhelmed by surfactant-laden material. It is also important to look for additional cellular clues as other diseases such as leukemia, *Nocardia*, and *Pneumocystis* are associated with PAP. The additional benefit of BAL in this disease is that it actually serves as the treatment of choice for the disease.

Interstitial Lung Disease

BAL may sometimes be helpful to differentiate some of the many causes of diffuse interstitial disease seen on chest imaging; however, it is generally not diagnostic as a stand-alone test. It is also used to monitor the degree of inflammation and therapeutic response. The cell count and differential from the fluid in some instances can be used to gauge disease activity.

In idiopathic pulmonary fibrosis with the histopathologic makeup of usual interstitial pneumonia (UIP), BAL will demonstrate a significant increase in neutrophils. The presence of eosinophils in this setting may be a marker for a less favorable response to antiinflammatory medications. It has also been reported that the presence of lymphocytes may assist in distinguishing nonspecific interstitial pneumonia from UIP.

Eosinophilic Lung Disease

The cell count and differential obtained from BAL are helpful in creating the differential diagnosis of the pulmonary diseases that are associated with >25% eosinophils in BAL. Some of these may include Churg–Strauss syndrome, allergic bronchopulmonary aspergillosis, drug-induced lung disease, and idiopathic pulmonary fibrosis. Acute and chronic eosinophilic pneumonia are included in this list and often have eosinophil counts in BAL that exceed 40%.

Alveolar Hemorrhage

Hemosiderin-laden macrophages indicate hemorrhage. The use of bronchoscopic assessment plays a dual role in identifying the presence of hemorrhage and in localizing the site of hemorrhage in focal radiographic disease. Localization of the hemorrhage may assist either the interventional radiologist or thoracic surgeon regarding the possibility of vascular embolization or resection, respectively.

Langerhans Cell Histiocytosis

This disease entity with primarily upper lobe involvement can be identified with BAL analysis with the use of the following methods: S-100 protein staining, OKT-6 (CD-1 antigen) monoclonal antibody staining, and electron microscopy demonstrating the presence of Birbeck granules. The latter is not often performed because of cost. It is also important to mention that, although BAL can be diagnostic, studies have shown that these findings can be seen in groups of patients with other types of interstitial lung disease and in smokers; therefore, a conclusive diagnosis may ultimately require a lung biopsy.

Sarcoidosis

The predominance of activated T helper cells producing an increased CD4-to-CD8 ratio of $\geq$4:1 demonstrates a positive predictive value of 94% for sarcoidosis. If the CD4-to-CD8 ratio is decreased, <1:1, the negative predictive value is 100%. As an adjunct to endobronchial and transbronchial biopsies, these BAL findings enhance the diagnostic sensitivity. BAL is not considered a sole diagnostic procedure as the presence of noncaseating granulomas is necessary for a confirmatory diagnosis. Additionally, there is no clear consensus as to the role of BAL assessment for following disease activity in these patients.

Berylliosis

The CD4-to-CD8 ratio in BAL fluid in this disease is also increased as seen in sarcoidosis. BAL cells are used in beryllium lymphocyte transformation testing to assist in this diagnosis.

Asbestosis

The finding of asbestos bodies in BAL indicates exposure but does not directly correlate with the presence of disease. This, however, may be helpful in identifying occupational exposure and those who may be at increased risk for asbestosis.

Hypersensitivity Pneumonitis

A helpful feature of BAL in this disease is the decreased CD4-to-CD8 ratio of <1:1 caused by the increased presence of suppressor T cells.

Drug-Induced Lung Diseases

Generally, this group of diseases demonstrates an increase in both lymphocytes and eosinophils in BAL fluid. Amiodarone demonstrates features of foamy macrophages because of phospholipid accumulation. There will be the presence of amorphous granular extracellular material that needs to be distinguished from alveolar proteinosis and *Pneumocystis*. The presence of these cellular findings in the patient on amiodarone serves as a marker for exposure, but the findings need to be correlated with radiographic and physiologic changes to define true amiodarone-related lung disease.

Malignancy

The diagnostic yield for malignancy with BAL can be 69% or greater in the presence of visible endobronchial disease. BAL is considered a highly effective method to obtain cytologic proof of bronchial carcinoma. BAL is often recommended to be performed prior to biopsies to reduce the obscuration of diagnostic cytologic cells by erythrocytes. Atypical cells can be seen in the setting of acute inflammation and should be interpreted with caution and in the clinical context of the patient.

ENDOBRONCHIAL BRUSHING

Brushings can be obtained for microbiologic analysis or to assist in the diagnosis of malignancy. In the setting of lung cancer and in the presence of endobronchial disease, the diagnosis has been confirmed in 50%–90%. The overall sensitivity has been reported as 65% with a specificity of 98%. Studies have also indicated that obtaining a brush sample along with other washings or biopsy is cost effective and generally safe. Complications of endobronchial brushing include bleeding, and it is best avoided in the irreversibly coagulopathic patient. Interestingly, brushings can result in as much bleeding as biopsies can. Topical epinephrine 1 to 2 mL at (1:10,000 dilution) can be instilled through the working channel to assist with local vasoconstriction along with iced saline to reduce local hemorrhage prior to brushing. There is a selection of brushes (3-mm and 7-mm bristles) that can be used for cytology and for microbiologic specimen collection (Figure 9.4). The brush should be kept within its protective sheath while it is passed through the working bronchoscopic channel, then directed to the target site, as an assistant

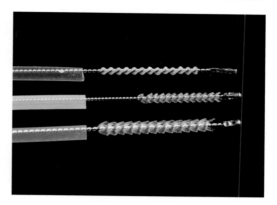

FIGURE 9.4 Bronchial brushes of varying sizes for microbiologic and cytologic evaluation.

advances the brush out approximately 3 cm or so from the bronchoscope. Vigorous brush strokes are then applied to the lesion. Communication to the assistant to bring the brush into its sheath when specimens have been retrieved should occur before the sheath and brush are pulled back through the working channel. Distal bronchial brushings or transbronchial brushings are usually performed with fluoroscopic guidance so as to avoid breaching the pleura and potentially causing a pneumothorax.

PSB in VAP

The advantage of using a PSB is the ability to maintain sterility and avoid contamination of the brush while traversing the proximal tracheobronchial tree. Not only is this brush safely encased in its protective sheath, there is a biodegradable plug at the distal end that is ejected when the brush is advanced in the desired location within the airway. Make sure to advance the entire device 3 cm or so beyond the distal tip of the bronchoscope into the desired airway and then push the brush out into the secretions. Retract the brush into the inner sheath, which in turn is retracted into the outer sheath and then removed from the bronchoscope. Wipe the distal part of the catheter with 70% alcohol, advance the brush component, and cut with sterile scissors into at least 1 mL of nonbacteriostatic saline. Request quantitative cultures. The specificity of this technique is reported as 70%. Interestingly, when this technique is compared with "blind" bronchial brush and BAL for VAP, there is no significant advantage in diagnostic yield between any of these. All are considered reliable alternatives. The quantitative culture analysis defines VAP with PSB as 1000 cfu/mL or 100–1000 cfu/mL in the presence of a strong clinical suspicion.

ENDOBRONCHIAL BIOPSY

The role for EBBX to obtain diagnostic material is best noted in malignancy, sarcoidosis, and tuberculosis. Endoscopically visible lesions understandably have a diagnostic yield in malignancy of >80%. In a review of 30 studies, the highest diagnostic yield for malignancy was with EBBX in visible disease as compared with cytology brushings followed by BWs. The diagnosis of sarcoidosis by this technique increased the yield of bronchoscopy by 20% and provided diagnostic tissue in 30% of patients with sarcoidosis even in the setting of normal-appearing airways. The role in chronic rejection in lung transplantation patients appears to be complementary to those of BAL and transbronchial biopsy.

The technique for EBBX depends on the location of the lesion relative to the airway wall or bifurcation of the airways. A "straight-on" approach is used with the biopsy forceps by use

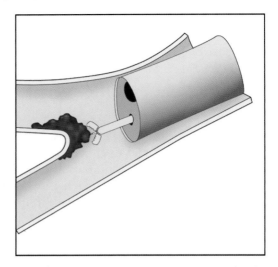

FIGURE 9.6 "Straight-on" approach at bronchial bifurcation with biopsy forceps with needle. (Illustration by Carla Lamb and Vinald Francis.)

of either cup or alligator biopsy forceps with or without a needle in a lesion that is at an airway bifurcation (Figures 9.5 and 9.6). Maintaining the bronchoscope close to the actual distal biopsy forceps and using them as one unit can provide the added leverage needed to push into the lesion to obtain a deeper core sample. If the lesion is parallel along the airway wall, then a more angular approach (preferably with the forceps with a needle) would allow for a more anchored position (Figure 9.7). It is advisable to take three to six biopsies in the same location to obtain the more central aspect of the lesion, as the surface cells may represent cellular edema and necrosis and not be diagnostic. To gain access to diagnostic cellular material, a 19- or 21-gauge needle can be directed into the core of the endobronchial lesion or where extrinsic compression of the airway wall is visible. Other variables such as lesion size, location of the lesion (tracheal or bronchial), vascularity, and submucosal versus polypoid or pedunculated lesions play a part in the clinician's approach to biopsy. A polypoid lesion may permit the use of an electrocautery snare (Figure 9.8) to lasso the lesion, apply heat, remove the lesion completely by removing it at its base, then retrieving it with biopsy forceps or a foreign body retrieval basket from the airway.

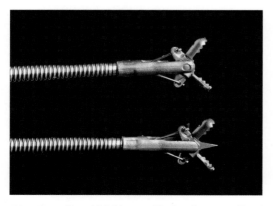

FIGURE 9.5 Bronchial biopsy alligator forceps without (*top*) and with (*bottom*) needle.

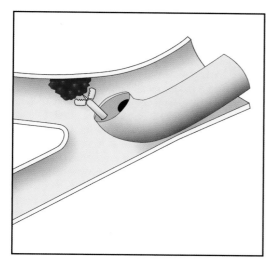

FIGURE 9.7 Angular side wall approach for endobronchial biopsy using needle to anchor the biopsy forceps to the tumor. (Illustration by Carla Lamb and Vinald Francis.)

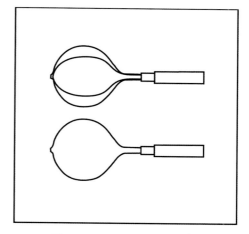

FIGURE 9.8 Electrocautery snares that can be used for biopsy in polypoid endobronchial lesions. (Illustration by Carla Lamb and Vinald Francis.)

If an airway lesion appears vascular or large in size where there is potential for significant bleeding or airway obstruction during EBBX, there are procedural strategies that might enhance patient safety. The use of topical epinephrine and iced saline instilled prior to the biopsy may reduce bleeding. Specifically, there should be consideration for rigid bronchoscopy with coagulation of the lesion with laser ablation, electrocautery, or cryotherapy prior to the biopsy.

ADVANCES IN BRONCHOALVEOLAR LAVAGE AND BRONCHIAL BRUSH IN LUNG CANCER

Two diagnostic tests continue to hold promise in early detection and diagnosis of lung cancer, especially in cases in which cytologic evaluation alone may be equivocal.

Airway epithelial gene expression can detect specific pattern changes in gene expression even while the airways appear grossly normal. This method can aid in the diagnosis of cancer and detect persons at risk for cancer caused by dysplastic degeneration as seen in smokers. Our institution found that endobronchial brushings of normal-appearing large airway epithelial cells,

when collected and analyzed with gene expression microarray, expressed an 80-gene biomarker that distinguished smokers with and without lung cancer. Ninety percent sensitivity was confirmed for Stage 1 lung cancer when patterns were reviewed.

Multitarget fluorescence in situ hybridization (FISH) is used for assessing and distinguishing reactive from malignant cells in patients with equivocal cytology. This technique detects chromosome-specific changes in interphase nuclei that allow direct cellular examination. The sensitivity is reported as 79%, specificity as 100%, and positive predictive value as 100%, with a 74% negative predictive value. This technique could be used in BWs, BALs, and brushings. FISH was more sensitive in individuals with non-small cell lung carcinoma and central tumors, and was also found to be more sensitive than conventional cytology from washings or brushings in the detection of lung cancer.

CONCLUSION

Although some of the procedures discussed here can be diagnostic individually for a variety of diseases, they are often used collectively to improve overall yield. As part of good preprocedural planning, the clinician should keep in mind the following:

- Carefully screen patients prior to the procedure for safety and ability to tolerate the anticipated diagnostic studies. Correct coagulopathies when brushes or biopsies are planned.
- Create a differential diagnosis to anticipate the volume of specimen required for desired testing.
- Be knowledgeable of the particular tests required.
- Have a strategy of collection anatomically based on chest imaging.
- Communicate to the bronchoscopy team these anticipated studies to ensure that proper specimen media are readily available.
- Communicate to microbiology and cytopathology the history and differential diagnosis to increase the level of awareness of specific disease entities.
- Recognize the diagnostic strengths and limits of each of these diagnostic procedures.

SUGGESTED READINGS

American Thoracic Society. Clinical role of bronchoalveolar lavage in adults with pulmonary disease. *Am Rev Respir Dis.* 1990;142:481–486.

American Thoracic Society; Infectious Diseases Society of America. Guidelines for the management of adults with hospital-acquired ventilator-associated and health care-associated pneumonia. *Am J Respir Crit Care Med.* 2005;171:388–416.

Boersma WG, Erjavec Z, Van Der Werf TS, et al. Bronchoscopic diagnosis of pulmonary infiltrates in granulocytopenic patients with hematologic malignancies: BAL versus PSB and PBAL. *Respir Med.* 2007;101:317–325.

British Thoracic Society Bronchoscopy Guidelines Committee. British Thoracic Society guidelines on diagnostic flexible bronchoscopy. *Thorax.* 2001;56(Suppl 1):1–21.

Brown M, Varia H, Davidson RN, Wall R, Pasvol G. Prospective study of sputum induction, gastric washing, and bronchoalveolar lavage for the diagnosis of pulmonary tuberculosis in patients who are unable to expectorate. *Clin Infect Dis.* 2007;44:1415–1420.

The Canadian Critical Care Trials Group. A randomized trial of diagnostic techniques for ventilator-associated

pneumonia. *N Engl J Med.* 2006;355(25):2619–2630.

Chastre J, Combes A, Luyt C. The invasive quantitative diagnosis of ventilator-associated pneumonia. *Respir Care.* 2005;50(6):797–812.

Cole P, Turton C, Lanyon H, Collins J. Bronchoalveolar lavage for preparation of free lung cells: technique and complications. *Br J Dis Chest.* 1980;74:273–278.

Costabel U, Hunninghake GW. ATS/ERS/WASOG statement on sarcoidosis. *Eur Respir J.* 1999;14:735–737.

Costabel U, Uzaslan E, Guzman J. Bronchoalveolar lavage in drug-induced lung disease. *Clin Chest Med.* 2004;25:25–35.

Fagon JY. Diagnosis and treatment of ventilator-associated pneumonia: fiberoptic bronchoscopy with bronchoalveolar lavage is essential. *Semin Respir Crit Care Med.* 2006;27(1):34–44.

Feller-Kopman D, Ernst A. The role of bronchoalveolar lavage in the immunocompromised host. *Semin Respir Infect.* 2003;18(2):87–94.

Fujitani S, Yu VL. Diagnosis of ventilator-associated pneumonia: focus on nonbronchoscopic techniques (nonbronchoscopic bronchoalveolar lavage, including mini-BAL, blinded protected specimen brush, and blinded bronchial sampling) and endotracheal aspirates. *J Intensive Care Med.* 2006;21:17–21.

Grossman RF, Fein A. Evidence-based assessment of diagnostic tests for ventilator-associated pneumonia. *Chest.* 2000;117:177–181.

Halling KC, Rickman OB, Kipp BR, Harwood AR, Doerr CH, Jett JR. A comparison of cytology and fluorescence in situ hybridization for the detection of lung cancer in bronchoscopic specimens. *Chest.* 2006;130:694–701.

Karahalli E, Yilmaz A, Turker H. Usefulness of various diagnostic techniques during fiberoptic bronchoscopy of endoscopically visible lung cancer: should cytologic examinations be performed routinely? *Respiration.* 2001;68:611–614.

King TE. Handling and analysis of bronchoalveolar lavage specimens. In: Baughman, RP, ed. *Bronchoalveolar Lavage.* St Louis: Mosby Year Book; 1991: 3–25.

Klech H, Pohl W, European Society of Pneumonology Task Group on BAL. Technical recommendations and guidelines for bronchoalveolar lavage (BAL). *Eur Respir J.* 1989;2:561–585.

Lam B, Wong MP, Ooi C, et al. Diagnostic yield of bronchoscopic sampling methods in bronchial carcinoma. *Respirology.* 2000;5:265–270.

Lamb CR, Lederman ER, Crum NF. Bronchoscopy: diagnostic and interventional approach in tropical pulmonary diseases. In: Sharma O, ed. *Tropical Lung Disease, 2nd ed.* New York: Taylor & Francis; 2006: 95–115.

Lee HS, Kwon SY, Kim DK, et al. Bronchial washing yield before and after forceps biopsy in patients with endoscopically visible lung cancers. *Respirology.* 2007;12:277–282.

Meersseman W, Lagrou K, Maertens J, et al. Galactomannan in bronchoalveolar lavage fluid: a tool for diagnosing aspergillosis in intensive care unit patients. *Am J Respir Crit Care Med.* 2008;177:27–34.

Michel F, Franceschini B, Berger P, et al. Early antibiotic treatment for BAL-confirmed ventilator-associated pneumonia. *Chest.* 2005;127:589–597.

Myer KC. The role of bronchoalveolar lavage in interstitial lung disease. *Clin Chest Med.* 2004;25:637–649.

Ost DE, Hall CS, Joseph G, et al. Decision analysis of antibiotic and diagnostic strategies in ventilator-associated pneumonia. *Am J Respir Crit Care Med.* 2003;168:1060–1067.

Pesci A, Majori M, Caminati A. Bronchoalveolar lavage in intensive care units. *Monaldi Arch Chest Dis.* 2004;61(1):39–43.

Rennard SI, Aalbers R, Bleecker E, et al. Bronchoalveolar lavage: performance, sampling procedure, processing and assessment. *Eur Respir J.* 1998;11(Suppl 26):13–15.

Reynolds HY. Use of bronchoalveolar lavage in humans–past necessity and future imperative. *Lung.* 2000;178:271–293.

Ryu YJ, Chung MP, Han J, et al. Bronchoalveolar lavage in fibrotic idiopathic interstitial pneumonias. *Respir Med.* 2007;101:655–660.

Savic S, Glatz K, Schoenegg R, et al. Multitarget fluorescence in situ hybridization elucidates equivocal lung cytology. *Chest.* 2006;129:1629–1635.

Travis WD, Colby TV, Koss MN, Rosado ML, Muller NL, King TE. Handling and analysis of bronchoalveolar lavage and lung specimens with approach to patterns of lung injury. *ARP Atlas, American Registry of Pathology.* 2007;1:17–42.

van der Drift MA, van der Wilt GJ, Thunnissen FB, Janssen JP. A prospective study of the timing and cost-effectiveness of bronchial washing during bronchoscopy for pulmonary malignant tumors. *Chest.* 2005;128:394–400.

Veeraaraghavan S, Latsi PI, Wells AU, et al. BAL findings in idiopathic nonspecific interstitial pneumonia and usual interstitial pneumonia. *Eur Respir J.* 2003;22:239–244.

10

TRANSBRONCHIAL LUNG BIOPSY

Scott Shofer and Momen M. Wahidi

INTRODUCTION

Transbronchial lung biopsy (TBB) is a safe and effective tool useful for the diagnosis of a wide variety of diffuse and focal pulmonary diseases. TBB is regularly performed by 69% of practicing physicians documented in a survey of 1,800 North American pulmonary and critical care physicians [1]. The procedure was first introduced by Andersen in 1965 for use via a rigid bronchoscope, and became more widely performed after it was adapted for use with the flexible bronchoscope in the early 1970s. This chapter describes the primary indications and contraindications to performing TBB during bronchoscopy, our approach to TBB, and methods to manage complications that may arise during or after the procedure.

INDICATIONS

Biopsy forceps commonly used for TBB via the flexible bronchoscope are generally of the order of 3 mm or smaller in any given dimension. Because of this restriction in size, tissue samples obtained via the transbronchial approach are generally 2–3 mm in any dimension. Despite the small size, TBB provides information regarding pathology that is located beyond the cartilaginous airways that may include elements of the small airways of the distal bronchial tree, the alveolar space, the vasculature, and lymphatic structures immediately surrounding the alveoli [2]. Pulmonary diseases that require examination of larger pieces of lung tissue to assess heterogeneity or homogeneity of different regions of the involved lung (such as many of the idiopathic interstitial lung diseases) are generally not amenable to diagnosis by TBB, so consideration of video-assisted thoracoscopic lung biopsy should be pursued for patients in whom these diseases are a strong consideration. With these limitations in mind, TBB is useful for the diagnosis of a variety of interstitial, infectious, and malignant pulmonary diseases (Table 10.1).

Interstitial Diseases

TBB has a high sensitivity for the diagnosis of sarcoidosis involving the lung. Even with Stage I disease, TBB may be positive in up to 50%–85% of patients undergoing this procedure [3], although yields are greater with increasing radiographic abnormality of the lung parenchyma. To optimize sampling of tissue for sarcoidosis, a minimum of four biopsies has been suggested to be collected before termination of the procedure [3]. TBB has a high yield in other interstitial lung diseases such as Langerhans cell histiocytosis, pulmonary alveolar proteinosis, lipoid pneumonia, eosinophilic pneumonia, and drug-induced pneumonitis [2].

Table 10.1. *Indications for TBB*

Sarcoidosis
Langerhans cell histiocytosis
Pulmonary alveolar proteinosis
Lipoid pneumonia
Eosinophilic pneumonia
Drug-induced pneumonitis
Pulmonary infiltrates in the
  immunocompromised host
Pulmonary carcinomatosis
Lymphangitic malignancy

Infectious Diseases

Diagnosis of infectious pulmonary disease in the immunocompromised host is a common indication for TBB. Sensitivity for infectious organisms ranges from 81% to 90% [4]. Although bronchoalveolar lavage (BAL) is often as efficacious as TBB in detecting infectious organisms in immunocompromised patients, in most series there are a small number of patients in whom the diagnosis is made by TBB but missed with BAL. In addition, compared with BAL, TBB enhances diagnostic yield for noninfectious etiologies in immunocompromised patients (an increase in yield from 31% to 40.4%, respectively) [5].

Infections with *Pneumocystis jiroveci* deserve special comment. BAL generally has excellent sensitivity for *Pneumocystis* infection in the patient with advanced HIV/AIDS, particularly when combined with immunofluorescent monoclonal antibody staining [6]. Additionally, when multilobar, site-directed BAL is performed, diagnostic yield is comparable to the yield obtained when TBB is added to the procedure even in the presence of pentamidine prophylaxis [6]. However, the sensitivity of BAL in immunocompromised hosts without HIV/AIDS may be lower. Addition of TBB to the diagnosis of *Pneumocystis* pneumonia in patients with cancer, bone marrow transplantation, or pharmacologic immunosuppression increases the diagnostic sensitivity from 82% to 92% [7].

Neoplastic Diseases

TBB is commonly used for the diagnosis of suspicious pulmonary nodules and masses. Overall, the yield of TBB for peripheral lesions is 57% although the yield from a specific nodule is related to size, location, and number of pieces of tissue collected. Sensitivity increases with the size of the nodule in question, with a diagnosis obtained 34% of the time in nodules <2 cm and 63% in nodules >2 cm. The presence of an airway leading to the nodule on thoracic computed tomography scan (positive bronchus sign) increases yield from 25% to 63% [8]. Diagnostic yield from pulmonary nodules increases with number of pieces of tissue collected. Popovich and colleagues [9] examined the effect of repeated sampling of peripheral pulmonary nodules by TBB. The initial biopsy had a sensitivity of 45%, which increased to 70% by the sixth sample. The authors noted that sensitivity continued to increase with repeated sampling, and as many as 10 pieces of tissue should be obtained to maximize diagnostic sensitivity of the procedure; however, this practice is not widely endorsed [9]. In malignancies with a diffuse distribution (such as bronchoalveolar cell carcinoma or lymphangitic tumor), sensitivity of TBB is generally good [10].

Lung Transplant Surveillance

TBB is the primary diagnostic procedure in evaluating the presence of allograft rejection in patients after lung transplantation [11]. Although surveillance strategies differ among various institutions, most institutions perform some form of TBB-based surveillance as well as diagnostic biopsies during periods of declining lung function in transplant recipients [11]. Sensitivity of TBB for allograft rejection has been reported to be as high as 94% when 10 or more pieces of tissue are collected [12], although most institutions do not regularly collect this many samples during surveillance bronchoscopies.

CONTRAINDICATIONS

Contraindications for TBB are similar to those for bronchoscopy in general. Absolute contraindications are few and include inability to provide informed consent, status asthmaticus, severe hypoxemia, and unstable cardiovascular conditions. Pulmonologists' perceptions of relative contraindications to TBB were examined during a recent survey of 158 North American respiratory physicians [13]. Physicians' opinions were obtained regarding the safety of TBB in the presence of thrombocytopenia, pulmonary hypertension, uremia, hypoxemia, and management of anticoagulant and antiplatelet medications.

Thrombocytopenia

Approximately 70% of the surveyed physicians felt that a platelet count of 50,000 was adequate to perform TBB safely [13]. Little data are available regarding bleeding complications from TBB in the thrombocytopenic patient. One series examined 24 patients with platelet count <60,000 and an average count of 30,000. Twenty of the 24 patients received prophylactic platelet transfusion prior to TBB with an incidence of significant bleeding in four patients, one of whom expired, and the remainder were self-limited [14]. Our practice has been to use a minimum platelet value of 50,000 when TBB is planned during the bronchoscopy. We have not experienced any life-threatening bleeding events related to thrombocytopenia in our practice using this criterion.

Pulmonary Hypertension

Sixty-five percent of surveyed physicians considered a mean pulmonary arterial pressure (MPAP) of >40 mm Hg a contraindication to TBB, whereas 25% responded that a MPAP between 25 and 40 mm Hg was a contraindication to TBB [13]. A single prospective study is available regarding TBB and pulmonary hypertension. This study examined 37 heart transplant recipients who had measurements of pulmonary pressures obtained within 72 hours of bronchoscopy. Moderate bleeding (defined as 25–100 cc of blood) was encountered in 15% of the 20 patients with MPAP >16 mmHg, whereas no significant bleeding occurred in the remaining patients. No

incidence of major hemorrhage occurred in any patients [15]. Current recommendations from the British Thoracic Society (BTS) suggest that caution should be observed in performance of TBB in patients with elevated pulmonary arterial pressures [10]. We have not established a pulmonary pressure at which TBB is contraindicated within our practice, and we assess each patient individually regarding the overall clinical scenario before we commit to performing TBB.

Uremia

The presence of uremia adversely affects platelet function, resulting in abnormal platelet aggregation and prolonged bleeding times [13], and potentially increasing the risk of significant hemorrhage in patients undergoing TBB. No studies that have rigorously examined the effect of uremia on bleeding complications in TBB currently exist. Some authors have suggested that the use of recombinant arginine vasopressin may decrease the extent of bleeding in uremic patients, although examination of the surgical literature has shown mixed results. The current practice at our institution is to give recombinant arginine vasopressin at a dose of 0.3 μg/kg intravenously to all lung transplant recipients with creatinine >2.5 mg/dL 30 minutes prior to bronchoscopy. Non-lung transplant patients generally do not receive arginine vasopressin, and we have not encountered noticeably increased rates of bleeding in these patients.

Hypoxemia

No level of oxygen supplementation is currently recognized to be an absolute contraindication to TBB, although 37% of surveyed pulmonologists indicated that an inspired oxygen requirement of >60% fraction of inspired oxygen (FiO_2) was a contraindication to TBB, whereas 36% of the respondents found no specific O_2 requirement a contraindication [13]. The BTS recommends supplying supplemental O_2 to keep blood oxygen saturations >90% to minimize the risk of cardiac arrhythmias during and following bronchoscopy [10]. Generally, we consider electively intubating patients for bronchoscopy when oxygen supplementation is >5 L/min via nasal cannula prior to performing TBB.

Anticoagulant and Antiplatelet Agents

Use of anticoagulants and antiplatelet agents is common among patients referred for bronchoscopy. No randomized trials exist regarding the use of warfarin in the setting of TBB. The BTS recommended holding warfarin for 3 days prior to bronchoscopy, or providing supplemental vitamin K prior to the procedure [10], and current recommendations suggest that an international normalized ratio of 1.5 is a safe level for most surgical procedures [16]. Patients anticoagulated with heparin should have this medication held for 6 hours prior to bronchoscopy and may be restarted 12 hours following the procedure. O'Donnell and colleagues [17] addressed the use of enoxaparin as a bridge for warfarin in patients scheduled for elective surgery. Ninety-four patients received a final dose of twice-daily enoxaparin at least 12 hours prior to surgery and were found to have persistently elevated anti-Xa levels at the time of surgery [17]. Based on these findings, it is our policy to hold therapeutically dosed enoxaparin for 24 hours prior to performing TBB, whereas enoxaparin dosed for deep vein thrombosis prophylaxis is held on the morning of the procedure.

Aspirin use was previously considered to be a contraindication to TBB; however, a large multicenter study has shown no difference in bleeding following TBB in 285 patients taking aspirin at the time of bronchoscopy compared with 932 patients not on aspirin [18]. Consequently, we do not have patients hold aspirin prior to TBB.

In a follow-up study examining the effect of the antiplatelet medication clopidogrel on incidence of bleeding during TBB, significant bleeding was increased to 89% compared with 3.4% in the control group [19]. In a small number of patients taking both aspirin and clopidogrel, the incidence of significant bleeding was 100% following TBB [19]. Given the relatively long half-life of clopidogrel, our current practice is to have patients discontinue clopidogrel a minimum of 5 days prior to undergoing bronchoscopy with TBB.

PROCEDURAL CONSIDERATIONS

TBB

TBB is most commonly performed via flexible bronchoscopy on patients under conscious sedation. Careful study of a prebronchoscopy CT scan is useful in determining the best pulmonary segment to access for biopsy. In diffuse pulmonary diseases, use of fluoroscopy is not necessary, although the risk of significant pneumothorax may be reduced (see below). In focal disease that is visible on chest x-ray, use of fluoroscopy during the procedure may significantly increase the diagnostic yield of the study.

After a careful airway examination is performed, the pulmonary segment of interest is intubated with the tip of the bronchoscope, and the pulmonary forceps are passed through the working channel of the bronchoscope. As the forceps are visualized entering the pulmonary subsegment, the fluoroscopy unit should be activated to visualize the forceps as they enter the distal segments of the lung (Figure 10.1). To take a biopsy of peripheral portions of the lung, the forceps should be gently advanced in the closed position until resistance is encountered (Figure 10.2). If fluoroscopy is used, the forceps may not appear to move very far within the lung if the direction of motion is within the plane of the imaging because of the two-dimensional nature of fluoroscopic imaging. If the fluoroscopy unit is equipped with a C-arm, the camera head may be rotated out of plane from the forceps to detect movement in the anterior–posterior direction relative to the patient. Next, the forceps are withdrawn approximately 1 cm, and the command is given to open the forceps jaws. The forceps are then advanced close to the area where resistance was encountered, and the forceps jaws are closed. With the fluoroscopy unit still activated, the

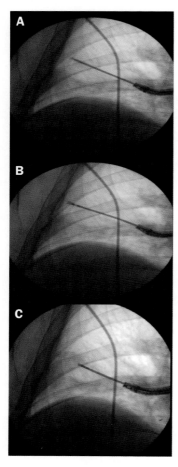

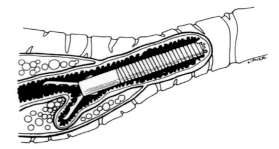

FIGURE 10.2. Artist's representation of forceps in the distal bronchus. The jaws of the forceps produce an invagination of the bronchial wall, resulting in sampling of both bronchial mucosa and alveolar tissue. (From Zavala DC. Transbronchial biopsy in diffuse lung disease. *Chest.* 1978;73:727–733, with permission)

FIGURE 10.1. Sequence of fluoroscopic images showing TBB from the right lung. Extension of the closed biopsy forceps to the periphery of the lung (A). Forceps opened and advanced to collect tissue (B). Forceps closed and partially withdrawn to collect the tissue sample (C). Note the subtle retraction of the underlying lung parenchyma by the forceps as the tissue sample is collected.

from the working channel of the bronchoscope, and the biopsy is placed in formalin.

Two schools of thought exist as to how best to manage the airway after a biopsy sample is collected. One school advocates use of the wedge technique, where the tip of the bronchoscope is lodged firmly (wedge position) in the airway subsegment that was sampled to monitor for bleeding. It is thought that leaving the bronchoscope wedged permits control of potential bleeding by continuous suctioning to remove extravasated blood, thereby preventing soiling of the remainder of the lung. Continuous suctioning also allows the operator to assess the quantity of bleeding present, and collapsing the distal airways produces a tamponade effect. When bleeding has slowed, the tip of the bronchoscope may be slowly withdrawn from the wedge position to allow observation of the bleeding segment and, if necessary, to facilitate repeating the wedge maneuver if the bleeding continues to be significant. The disadvantage of the wedge maneuver is that the bronchoscopist is not able to either visualize the airways because of blood obscuring the optics of the bronchoscope or to assess the effectiveness of the wedge in isolating the bleeding subsegment. In the alternative strategy, the tip of the bronchoscope is withdrawn from the subsegment of interest so that the bronchoscopist can watch for welling up of blood from the distal lung. Blood is suctioned with a

forceps are retracted with firm, continuous pressure to allow the biopsy specimen to be removed from the surrounding lung parenchyma. The lung parenchyma should be watched on the fluoroscopy monitor for retraction during the collection of the biopsy sample (Figure 10.1). If there is excessive resistance, or extensive retraction of the lung parenchyma during sampling, the forceps should be opened to release the lung tissue, and the biopsy procedure should be restarted. Once a sample is obtained, the forceps are removed back-and-forth motion to clear the airway and maintain vision. This suctioning permits a more global assessment of the extent of bleeding and potential seepage of blood into the other portions of the lung. There are currently no data to support the superiority of either approach. Our practice is to have novice bronchoscopists maintain wedge after each biopsy and use the observational technique after they have acquired more experience with the bronchoscope. Additional discussion of the management of bleeding complications is presented below.

Optimizing Biopsy Yield

Several studies have examined how best to enhance biopsy yield in terms of number of samples to be collected and characteristics of the collected specimens. As described above, the number of tissue pieces needed to optimize sensitivity is dependent on the underlying disease. Most studies report a range of 4–10 pieces of tissue to optimize sampling sensitivity [3,9,12], and the BTS guidelines on flexible bronchoscopy recommend four to six samples in patients with diffuse lung disease and seven to eight samples in patients with focal lung disease [10]. Our practice is to obtain a minimum of six tissue pieces of a minimum size of 1–2 mm in the long axis for patients with either focal or diffuse lung disease.

Several studies have examined the optimal size of biopsy forceps for performing TBB. No clear difference has been established regarding size of tissue samples or diagnostic sensitivity between large and small forceps, although one study using large, alligator-type forceps showed lower yields compared with those of large or small forceps. The lower yield was attributed to difficulty in passing the larger forceps past the various subcarinae of the small airways [20,21]. A third study examined the size and quality of tissue samples obtained with a small round cup, medium oval cup, or large, round-cup forceps. Tissue sample sizes were equal when the medium or large forceps were used, and larger in size than those obtained with the small forceps. However, the quality of the samples was greater when the oval

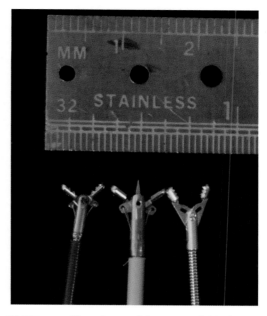

FIGURE 10.3. Three types of forceps available for use with the flexible bronchoscope. *Right to left*: small forceps with teeth; large, smooth-cupped forceps with center spike; and large forceps with teeth. The forceps fitted with a center spike are more commonly used for performing endobronchial biopsies.

forceps were used, revealing less crush artifact and more intact basement membrane on pathologic analysis [22]. An additional study examined the ability of physicians to predict the quality of TBB at the time of bronchoscopy. The authors found no significance to floating the tissue sample in formalin (suggesting alveolated tissue), and no ability of the physicians to predict the quality of the sample at the time the specimen was obtained. The authors did find that alligator forceps obtained larger samples compared with cup-type forceps of a similar size (3 mm), although the samples were graded for size with a technician's observation used as the assessment tool (as opposed to a microscopic measurement used in the other studies described above) [23]. Our practice is to use medium-sized oval cup forceps (Figure 10.3) for all of our TBBs because they do not entirely occlude the working channel of the bronchoscope while the forceps are extended, thereby permitting continued use of the working

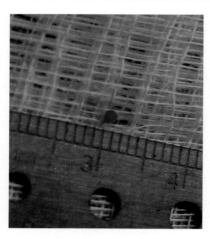

FIGURE 10.4. Representative TBB specimen. Note small size of tissue sample, approximately 1 mm in diameter.

channel for suctioning. Larger forceps show no clear advantage in biopsy quality, but do preclude effective suctioning while they are deployed (Figure 10.4).

After Procedure Care

Following bronchoscopy with TBB, patients should be observed in a recovery unit similar to that used by other patients receiving conscious sedation [10]. Given the increased risk of hemorrhage with TBB, we recommend that outpatients continue to hold their anticoagulants or antiplatelet agents until the morning following the procedure. Inpatients may resume anticoagulants such as heparin or enoxaparin 12 hours after the procedure.

COMPLICATIONS

Bronchoscopy with TBB is a safe procedure; however, complications do arise in 5%–9% of procedures [24]. Primary complications that arise with TBB are pneumothorax and hemorrhage. Pneumothorax occurs in 1%–6% of patients undergoing TBB [24,25]. Symptoms include chest pain, hemoptysis, and shortness of breath after the procedure. The need for chest radiography after TBB is controversial. In a single study examining

the incidence of pneumothorax after TBB, pneumothorax was identified in 10 of 259 nonlung transplant patients, 7 of whom developed symptoms suggestive of pneumothorax. The three patients who were asymptomatic had small pneumothoraces that did not require additional intervention, whereas 4 of the 7 symptomatic patients had large pneumothoraces that required chest tube insertion. Severity of symptoms coincided with size of pneumothorax. The authors concluded that routine radiography is not necessary after TBB in patients who are able to describe symptoms after biopsy [25]. The use of fluoroscopy during TBB has not been shown to reduce risk of pneumothorax [10], although a survey of 328 chest physicians in the United Kingdom showed a significantly lower incidence of reported pneumothorax requiring chest tube drainage in the past year for those who routinely used fluoroscopy [26]. No significant difference in the total number of pneumothoraces was noted between the two groups (0.86% vs. 1.15%) [26]. It is our practice to routinely use fluoroscopy during TBB and to perform a fluoroscopic screen for pneumothorax at the completion of the procedure. Chest x-rays are performed in all patients who develop symptoms of chest pain, increased shortness of breath, or unexplained hypoxia after the bronchoscopy.

Significant hemorrhage, defined as >50 mL of blood, is observed in 2%–9% of patients undergoing TBB [24]. No randomized studies have been published on the optimal management of hemorrhage related to TBB, although several recommendations have been proposed by recognized experts. Zavala [27] first described the wedge technique in 1976, whereby the tip of the bronchoscope is placed within the subsegment that is being biopsied. The forceps used for the biopsy are passed through the working channel of the bronchoscope and extended into the subsegment, and the biopsy is obtained. Afterward, the forceps are removed and the bronchoscope is left in position to isolate the subsegment and prevent the seepage of blood into the remainder of the bronchial tree. Blood is suctioned for a recommended period of 5 minutes to permit clotting, and the bronchoscope is cautiously withdrawn from the subsegment (so that it can be observed for further bleeding) [27]. As noted above, no data exist to suggest that the wedge technique decreases significant bleeding or related complications.

Additional therapeutic modalities that have been suggested include the use of iced saline administered via the working channel of the bronchoscope placed in the wedge position. Our practice is to give a 20-mL bolus of iced saline and withhold suctioning for several minutes to allow the cold fluid to induce local vasoconstriction. If the first bolus is unsuccessful, the fluid is suctioned and a second bolus is administered, repeating the observation period for several minutes. If this process is unsuccessful in controlling bleeding, 20 mL of 1:20,000 epinephrine is administered [10], and the patient is placed with the hemorrhaging lung down to prevent soiling of the uninvolved lung. Using these measures, the majority of hemorrhages related to TBB will be controlled. Occasionally, the bleeding may be severe enough to require placement of an endobronchial blocker.

CONCLUSIONS

TBB is a useful and safe diagnostic tool for the appropriately trained pulmonologist. A wide variety of inflammatory, malignant, and infectious pulmonary diseases are amenable to diagnosis by TBB and, in the diagnosis of pulmonary malignancies, TBB is the procedure of choice in the appropriate setting. Complications are rare and generally easily managed by the well-trained physician.

REFERENCES

1. Prakash UB, Offord KP, Stubbs SE. Bronchoscopy in North America: the ACCP survey. *Chest.* 1991;100:1668–1675.
2. Leslie KO, Gruden JF, Parish JM, Scholand MB. Transbronchial biopsy interpretation in the patient with diffuse parenchymal lung disease. *Arch Pathol Lab Med.* 2007;131:407–423.
3. Gilman MJ, Wang KP. Transbronchial lung biopsy in sarcoidosis: an approach to determine the optimal number of biopsies. *Am Rev Respir Dis.* 1980;122:721–724.
4. Matthay RA, Farmer WC, Odero D. Diagnostic fiberoptic bronchoscopy in the immunocompromised host with pulmonary infiltrates. *Thorax.* 1977;32:539–545.
5. Cazzadori A, DiPerri G, Todeschini G, et al. Transbronchial biopsy in the diagnosis of pulmonary infiltrates in immunocompromised patients. *Chest.* 1995;107:101–106.
6. Levine SJ, Kennedy D, Shelhamer JH, et al. Diagnosis of *Pneumocystis carinii* pneumonia by multiple lobe site-directed bronchoalveolar lavage with immunofluorescent monoclonal antibody staining in human immunodeficiency virus-infected patients receiving aerosolized pentamidine chemoprophylaxis. *Am Rev Respir Dis.* 1992;146:838–843.
7. Stover DE, Zaman MB, Hajdu SI, Lange M, Gold J, Armstrong D. Bronchoalveolar lavage in the diagnosis of diffuse pulmonary infiltrates in the immunosuppressed host. *Ann Intern Med.* 1984;101:1–7.
8. Naidich DP, Sussman R, Kutcher WL, Aranda CP, Garay SM, Ettenger NA. Solitary pulmonary nodules. CT-bronchoscopic correlation. *Chest.* 1988;93:595–598.
9. Popovich J Jr, Kvale PA, Eichenhorn MS, Radke JR, Ohorodnik JM, Fine G. Diagnostic accuracy of multiple biopsies from flexible fiberoptic bronchoscopy. A comparison of central versus peripheral carcinoma. *Am Rev Respir Dis.* 1982;125:521–523.
10. British Thoracic Society Bronchoscopy Guidelines Committee. British Thoracic Society guidelines on diagnostic flexible bronchoscopy. *Thorax.* 2001;56(Suppl 1):i1–i21.
11. Glanville AR. The role of bronchoscopic surveillance monitoring in the care of lung transplant recipients. *Semin Respir Crit Care Med.* 2006;27:480–491.
12. Scott JP, Fradet G, Smyth RL, et al. Prospective study of transbronchial biopsies in the management of heart-lung and single lung transplant patients. *J Heart Lung Transplant.* 1991;10:626–636.
13. Wahidi MM, Roca AT, Hollingsworth JW, Govert JA, Feller-Kopman D, Ernst A. Contraindications and safety of transbronchial lung biopsy via flexible bronchoscopy. *Respiration.* 2005;72:285–295.
14. Papin TA, Lynch JP III, Weg JG. Transbronchial biopsy in the thrombocytopenic patient. *Chest.* 1985;88:549–552.

15. Schulman LL, Smith CR, Drusin R, Rose EA, Enson Y, Reemtsma K. Utility of airway endoscopy in the diagnosis of respiratory complications of cardiac transplantation. *Chest.* 1988;93:960–967.

16. Kearon C, Hirsh J. Management of anticoagulation before and after elective surgery. *N Engl J Med.* 1997;336:1506–1511.

17. O'Donnell MJ, Kearon C, Johnson J, et al. Brief communication: Preoperative anticoagulant activity after bridging low-molecular-weight heparin for temporary interruption of warfarin. *Ann Intern Med.* 2007;146:184–187.

18. Herth FJ, Becker HD, Ernst A. Aspirin does not increase bleeding complications after transbronchial biopsy. *Chest.* 2002;122:1461–1464.

19. Ernst A, Eberhardt R, Wahidi M, Becker HD, Herth FJF. Effect of routine clopidogrel use on bleeding complications after transbronchial biopsy in humans. *Chest.* 2006;129:734–737.

20. Loube DI, Johnson JE, Wiener D, Anders GT, Blanton HM, Hayes JA. The effect of forceps size on the adequacy of specimens obtained by transbronchial biopsy. *Am Rev Respir Dis.* 1993;148:1411–1413.

21. Smith LS, Seaquist M, Schillaci RF. Comparison of forceps used for transbronchial lung biopsy: bigger may not be better. *Chest.* 1985;87:574–576.

22. Aleva RM, Kraan J, Smith M, ten Hacken NH, Postma DS, Timens W. Quantity and morphology of bronchial biopsy specimens taken by forceps of three sizes. *Chest.* 1998;113:182–185.

23. Curley FJ, Johal JS, Burke ME, Fraire AE. Transbronchial lung biopsy: can specimen quality be predicted at the time of biopsy? *Chest.* 1998;113:1037–1041.

24. Pue C, Pacht E. Complications of fiberoptic bronchoscopy at a university hospital. *Chest.* 1995;107:430–432.

25. Izbicki G, Shitrit D, Yarmolovsky A, et al. Is routine chest radiography after transbronchial biopsy necessary?: A prospective study of 350 cases. *Chest.* 2006;129:1561–1564.

26. Smyth CM, Stead RJ. Survey of flexible fibreoptic bronchoscopy in the United Kingdom. *Eur Respir J.* 2002;19:458–463.

27. Zavala DC. Pulmonary hemorrhage of fiberoptic transbronchial biopsy. *Chest.* 1976;70:584–588.

11

TRANSBRONCHIAL NEEDLE ASPIRATION

William Fischer and David Feller-Kopman

INTRODUCTION

Transbronchial needle aspiration (TBNA) is a technique that has revolutionized the diagnosis of mediastinal pathology by enabling intrathoracic nodal sampling in a minimally invasive manner. The sampling of paratracheal masses using an esophageal varix needle passed through a rigid bronchoscope was initially described by Ko-Pen Wang in 1978. The following year Oho and colleagues created a needle that could be passed through a flexible bronchoscope, thus ushering in a novel modality for sampling intrathoracic lymph nodes without surgical intervention. Over the last 30 years, the technique of TBNA has been relatively unchanged, although the indications for TBNA have expanded to include sampling of hilar lymph nodes, submucosal disease, visible endobronchial lesions, as well as peripheral nodules. The recent development of advanced imaging such as computed tomography (CT) fluoroscopy, electromagnetic navigation, and endobronchial ultrasound (EBUS) now allows real-time visualization of lymph node sampling. Because of these advances, TBNA has emerged as the first line of intrathoracic lymph node sampling for the diagnosis, staging, and prognosis of bronchogenic carcinoma, sarcoidosis, and even infectious diseases.

Bronchogenic carcinoma is the leading cause of cancer death in both men and women in the United States as well as in several other countries. Therapeutic options and prognoses are heavily dependent on accurate staging, and nodal staging is a key component of determining overall clinical stage (Figure 11.1). Non-invasive radiologic staging is suboptimal with sensitivities ranging from 51% to 74%. Additionally, because radiologic staging has been demonstrated to differ markedly from pathologic staging, the American Thoracic Society (ATS), European Respiratory Society (ERS), and European Society of Cardiothoracic Surgery all recommend that pathologic evaluation of the mediastinum be obtained in all patients prior to surgical resection of lung cancer. Mediastinoscopy has long been the gold standard for obtaining tissue, with sensitivities and specificities of 80%–90% and 100%, respectively. Comparatively, the overall sensitivity of TBNA is 78%. Despite a high specificity (99%), TBNA is limited by a higher false-negative rate compared with that of mediastinoscopy (28% vs. 11%). The yield with TBNA has been associated with tumor cell type (small cell > non-small cell > lymphoma), lymph node size, and lymph node location. EBUS-TBNA has been shown to have a sensitivity and specificity of approximately 94% and 100%, respectively, and its yield may be independent of lymph node size and location. Nonetheless, if TBNA is nondiagnostic, surgical sampling

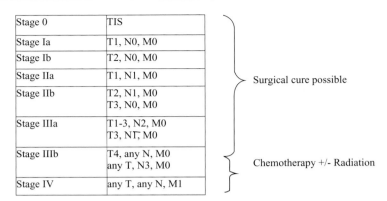

Stage 0	TIS
Stage Ia	T1, N0, M0
Stage Ib	T2, N0, M0
Stage IIa	T1, N1, M0
Stage IIb	T2, N1, M0 T3, N0, M0
Stage IIIa	T1-3, N2, M0 T3, N1, M0
Stage IIIb	T4, any N, M0 any T, N3, M0
Stage IV	any T, any N, M1

Surgical cure possible

Chemotherapy +/- Radiation

FIGURE 11.1. Possible treatment options for patients with non-small cell lung cancer.

is still recommended to rule out mediastinal nodal involvement. As a minimally invasive procedure, TBNA offers the significant benefit of fewer complications and has been demonstrated to preclude surgery in as many as 66% of patients.

TBNA can also be used for peripheral parenchymal opacities. For peripheral lung cancer, TBNA has been shown to have a higher diagnostic yield than brushing or transbronchial biopsy. Peripheral TBNA is the exclusive diagnostic modality in up to 35% of cases, can obtain diagnostic tissue in up to 76% of cases, and significantly increases the yield when combined with other modalities used to sample peripheral opacities such as bronchoalveolar lavage (BAL), brushing, and/or transbronchial biopsy.

The major limitation of TBNA is that it remains an underused technique. Two recent surveys have found that only 12% of pulmonologists routinely used TBNA in the evaluation of malignant disease. This likely results from fears of not obtaining adequate tissue, fears of causing damage to the bronchoscope, as well as inadequate training during fellowship. Among these reasons, lack of training is likely the foremost reason for the underuse of TBNA in clinical practice.

ANATOMY

It is crucial that the bronchoscopist become an expert in airway anatomy, and there are several excellent chapters and texts to assist with this process. In addition to the upper airway and the segmental anatomy of the lungs, it is essential to have a comprehensive understanding of the anatomy external to the airway, primarily the intrathoracic vessels and lymph nodes. To maximize the sensitivity of TBNA, Wang proposed a staging system and anatomic guide for needle placement as defined by the CT scan and bronchoscopic imaging. Although extremely useful to the bronchoscopist, this lymph node map has one important limitation in that the nodal stations do not correspond exactly to those used by radiologists and thoracic surgeons. For example, in the system proposed by Wang, the left paratracheal station (4L) is also called the "aortic-pulmonary window." On the ATS/ERS lymph node map, however, the aortic-pulmonary window actually refers to station 5 and 6 nodes, which lie on the lateral side of the ligamentum arteriosum, and are therefore inaccessible by TBNA. As communication with our colleagues is essential, we recommend using the system proposed by the ATS and ERS (Figure 11.2). That way, when the surgeons and radiologists refer to a left paratracheal lymph node (station 4L), everyone will be on the same page.

To improve one's yield, Wang suggested flipping the right and left CT images to help visualize the anatomic location of the lymph node relative to the airway during the procedure. Virtual bronchoscopy, by making the airway wall translucent and highlighting the target lymph

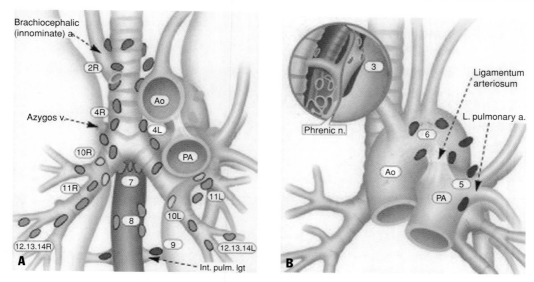

FIGURE 11.2. ATS/ERS lymph node map (From: *Am J Respir Crit Care Med.* 1997; 156:320).

node, may also aid the bronchoscopist by having the visual of the relevant anatomy in the "mind's eye" during the procedure. The major drawback to these techniques is that the bronchoscopist is still required to mentally transpose the images during the procedure, and remains uncertain as to final needle position. Failure to place the needle directly into the lesion remains the leading cause of a lower yield on biopsy. Among lymph nodes of equivalent size, right paratracheal (4R) and subcarinal (7) stations have been shown to have a higher diagnostic yield than nodes in other stations. As such, these should be the first nodal stations attempted by novice operators.

EQUIPMENT

Although there are many different types of TBNA needles available for use, they can be divided into two broad categories: histology (19-gauge) and cytology (22-gauge) needles. Some histology needles have an inner 21-gauge needle and an outer 19-gauge needle, whereas others are a single 19-gauge needle. There has never been, and likely will never be, a study showing that

one particular needle is better than another. Therefore, the bronchoscopist should familiarize him- or herself with one particular histology needle and one particular cytology needle.

Schenk and colleagues have shown that the 19-gauge needle provides a higher diagnostic yield as compared with that of the 22-gauge needle when used for lung cancer staging. All transbronchial needles consist of (1) a distal retractable sharp beveled needle, (2) a flexible catheter with a metal hub at the distal end, (3) a proximal control device used to manipulate the needle, and (4) a proximal side port through which suction can be applied.

TECHNIQUE

When used for the staging of non-small cell lung cancer (NSCLC), it is of utmost importance to avoid false-positive results, which would have the clinical effect of upstaging a patient, and potentially precluding curative surgery. For this reason, TBNA should be the first procedure performed during the bronchoscopy, and the lymph node station that would place the patient at the highest stage should be sampled first. For example, in the

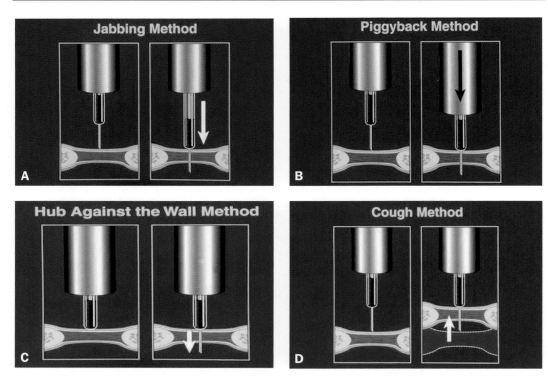

FIGURE 11.3. Common techniques for transbronchial needle aspiration. From: Dasgupta A, Mehta A, Wang KP. Transbronchial needle aspiration. *Semin Respir Crit Care Med.* 1997;18:571–581.

case of a patient with a T2 lesion in the left upper lobe, with adenopathy in stations 4L, 4R, and 7, the 4R node should be sampled first, as it would be considered N3, and therefore make the patient stage IIIb, and therefore not a surgical candidate. If the bronchoscopist attempted a BAL, brush, and transbronchial biopsy of the left upper lobe lesion first, the working channel of the bronchoscope could become contaminated and provide a false-positive result for subsequent TBNAs.

The Golden Rule of TBNA is "never advance the catheter in the bronchoscope with the needle out." A corollary to this rule is that the bronchoscopist is only as good as his or her support staff. It is essential to train your assistant prior to performing the procedure to be sure that he or she knows how to operate the needle. When the bronchoscope is in the desired location, the operator should keep the tip of the bronchoscope midline in the airway and advance the needle assembly

through the working channel of the bronchoscope, making sure that the needle is retracted into the metal needle hub. After the catheter tip is visible within the bronchial lumen, the needle is advanced and locked into place. If at any time prior to needle insertion into the airway, the needle tip is *not* visible, it should immediately be retracted by the assistant. Once the bronchoscope is at the level of the target lymph node, the bronchoscope is flexed up so that the needle tip is as perpendicular to the airway wall as possible. Passage of the needle through the airway wall can occur in one of four methods, as described by Dasgupta and Mehta (Figure 11.3).

Jabbing Method

This method begins by retracting the catheter and extended needle so that only the tip of the needle is visible, again being careful not to withdraw the needle tip into the bronchoscope. The bronchoscope is flexed to position the needle perpendicular to the airway wall, and the needle is then advanced while the bronchoscope is held stationary.

Piggyback Method

As with the jabbing method, the extended needle is withdrawn such that only the tip of the needle is visible. Force is then applied to the bronchoscope and the needle–catheter apparatus until the needle penetrates the target lymph node. The bronchoscope thus provides a rigid support to the flexible needle to penetrate the bronchial wall.

Hub Against the Wall Method

This method begins with placement of the catheter hub against the airway wall adjacent to the target lymph node with the needle retracted in the hub. The needle is then deployed directly into the target tissue.

Cough Method

With the needle exposed through the catheter, it is positioned against the target lymph node. The patient is then instructed to cough, thereby pushing the bronchial wall against the needle.

In our practice, we typically start with the jabbing method; however, certain circumstances may require other techniques, and we will often use more than one method in any given procedure.

When in the target lesion, suction should be applied to ensure that the needle has not passed into a vessel. If blood is aspirated, suction should be released, the needle retracted, and another location selected. If blood is not aspirated, the needle should be passed in and out of the target. The syringe should then be disconnected from the catheter, the bronchoscope placed in a neutral position, and the needle withdrawn back into the catheter. The catheter is then removed in a single smooth motion from the bronchoscope.

Although one study suggests that, for NSCLC, there is diminishing return after seven passes at a given lymph node, a more recent study by Diacon's group suggests that this may occur after four needle passes. As stated above, factors such as underlying tumor histology, lymph node size, and station may influence these recommendations.

SPECIMEN PROCESSING AND INTERPRETATION

All material from the biopsy should be processed to maximize the yield from the procedure. A sample from a 19-gauge needle can be sent in formalin as a "core biopsy" to surgical pathology or be processed by cytopathology. Samples from a 22-gauge needle, however, should all be processed by cytopathology. It is important to talk to the surgical and cytopathology departments at one's institution to determine how they prefer their specimens. Some institutions have rapid on-site evaluation (ROSE) and may prefer that the specimen be placed directly on a glass slide for immediate staging, whereas other institutions prefer that the material for cytologic analysis be placed in CytoLyt or another medium. Several studies have shown that the use of ROSE is associated with a reduction in the number of inadequate specimens. This may be less of an issue with the development of real-time imaging provided by EBUS, but we still feel that it is important to review the results from all cases. This serves to enhance one's technique and provide feedback as to what worked and what did not for a particular needle pass. A major caveat for ROSE is the potential for a false-positive result that leads to premature termination of the procedure. As such, it is crucial that the cytopathologists be experienced in interpreting TBNA and only state that they have an adequate tissue sample when they are confident.

As TBNA does not have a 100% negative predictive value, we do prefer the term "nondiagnostic" to "negative." This is an important concept to explain to the patient as well, as, if the TBNA does not provide an answer, it may be essential to take the next step, perhaps a mediastinoscopy, and obtain more tissue.

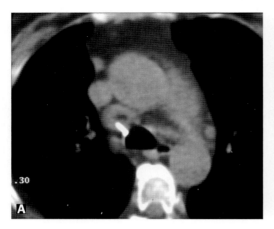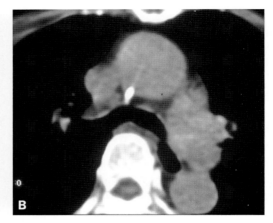

FIGURE 11.4. CTF showing **(A)** needle appropriately placed in station 4R node and **(B)** needle in aorta.

COMPLICATIONS

TBNA is perhaps the safest bronchoscopic procedure available, with an overall complication rate of 0.26%. There have been case reports of bleeding, infection, pneumothorax, and pneumomediastinum; however, serious adverse effects are much less frequent when compared with those from transbronchial biopsy or surgical biopsy.

Improving the Yield

Clearly, experience counts. In a recent study by Hsu and colleagues, the sensitivity of TBNA increased from 33% to 81% over a period of 3.5 years. To gain experience, we recommend a commitment to learning mediastinal anatomy, understanding the technique from a conceptual standpoint, practicing the procedure on either a simulator or other model to gain the psychomotor skills, and then performing the procedure on as many patients with mediastinal and hilar adenopathy as possible. Feedback is essential, and it is crucial to review all cytology/pathology samples and to try to reference each pass with the technique used to obtain the tissue. This is a key benefit that ROSE can provide during the learning curve of TBNA.

The use of 19-gauge histology needles has been shown to increase the yield when compared

with the use of cytology (22-gauge) needles, especially for nonmalignant disease. As above, we recommend that the operator become familiar with both a histology and a cytology needle. If the diagnosis leading the differential is not malignancy, the histology needle should be used.

The use of CT fluoroscopy (CTF) can be used to provide real-time confirmation of needle location. As opposed to standard fluoroscopy, which is typically used only in two dimensions, CT provides the ability to visualize the target in three dimensions and provides real-time three-dimensional confirmation of the appropriate (Figure 11.4A) and inappropriate (Figure 11.4B) biopsy sites. A study by Goldberg and colleagues analyzed data from 12 patients who underwent CTF-guided TBNA via a "quick-check" technique after having previously undergone nondiagnostic conventional BNA. A diagnosis was made in all patients, with a mean procedure time and number of aspirates similar to historical controls. Additionally, CTF confirmed that only 6 of the initial 18 (33%) needle passes were properly positioned within the target lymph node. With guidance, the rate of subsequent successful passes increased to 62%. Despite the fact that the TBNAs were performed by an experienced interventional pulmonologist, 42% of the needle insertions were not in the intended target. Six insertions (5.2%) were seen to have penetrated great vessels (four in the pulmonary artery, and one each in the left atrium and aorta); however, all of these were without complication.

Ernst's group went on to describe their results obtained by CTF in 32 patients with hilar and mediastinal adenopathy. As the yield with conventional TBNA is relatively high for nodes in the subcarinal and precarinal stations, patients with adenopathy in these areas were required to have a prior nondiagnostic TBNA to be included in the study. Adequate tissue was obtained in 28 patients (87.5%), and a specific diagnosis was made in 22 (68.8%). One patient had a false-negative CTF-guided TBNA. The authors conclude that, although CTF is not a substitute for good TBNA technique, it is an extremely helpful tool to improve the yield of TBNA in small and less accessible nodes.

EBUS is another important modality used to help improve accuracy of TBNA. Like CTF, EBUS has also been shown to significantly improve the yield of TBNA. Recently, a bronchoscope with a dedicated ultrasound probe and distinct working channel was developed (Olympus Corporation, Tokyo, Japan), and has the benefit of providing real-time guidance for TBNA of mediastinal and hilar lymph nodes, with excellent results. The sensitivity, specificity, and negative predictive value for EBUS-TBNA are 98.7%, 100%, and 97%, respectively. For lymphoma, EBUS-TBNA has been shown to have sensitivity, specificity, and negative predicative value of 91%, 100%, and 93%, respectively, despite the fact that the currently available needle for use in EBUS-TBNA is 22 gauge. Herth and colleagues have recently shown that, even in the presence of a radiographically normal mediastinum (as defined by no nodes >1 cm on CT), EBUS identified malignancy in nearly 20% of patients, and avoided surgery in 17%.

SUMMARY

Despite TBNA being available for nearly 30 years, it remains one of the most underused tools

of the pulmonologist. TBNA is an extremely safe procedure and should be routinely used to sample mediastinal and hilar lymph nodes, endobronchial lesions, as well as parenchymal opacities. EBUS-TBNA now allows real-time guidance of lymph nodes and may preclude the need for surgery in a significant number of patients. These new technologies, however, do not make one a better bronchoscopist; we therefore recommend dedicated training and continued practice.

SUGGESTED READINGS

American Thoracic Society and The European Respiratory Society. Pretreatment evaluation of non-small-cell lung cancer. *Am J Respir Crit Care Med.* 1997;156(1):320–332.

Becker HD. *Atlas of Bronchoscopy: Technique, Diagnosis, Differential Diagnosis, Therapy.* Philadelphia: BC Decker; 1991.

Cortese DA, Prakash UBS. Anatomy for the bronchoscopist. In: Prakash UBS, ed. *Bronchoscopy.* New York: Raven Press, Ltd.; 1994:13–42.

Dasgupta A, Mehta AC. Transbronchial needle aspiration. An underused diagnostic technique. *Clin Chest Med.* 1999;20(1):39–51.

Dasgupta A, Mehta A, Wang KP. Transbronchial needle aspiration. *Semin Respir Crit Care Med.* 1997;18:571–581.

Davenport RD. Rapid on-site evaluation of transbronchial aspirates. *Chest.* 1990;98(1):59–61.

De Leyn P, Lardinois D, Van Schil PE, Rami-Porta, R, Passlick, B, Zielinski, M, Waller, DA, Lerut, T, Weder, W. ESTS guidelines for preoperative lymph node staging for non-small cell lung cancer. *Eur J Cardiothorac Surg.* 2007;32(1):1–8.

Detterbeck FC, Jantz MA, Wallace M, Vansteenkiste, J, Silvestri G. Invasive mediastinal staging of lung cancer: ACCP evidence-based clinical practice guidelines (2nd ed.). *Chest.* 2007;132(3 Suppl):202S–220S.

Diacon AH, Schuurmans MM, Theron J, Brundyn K, Louw M, Wright CA, Bolliger CT. Transbronchial needle aspirates: how many passes per target site? *Eur Respir J.* 2007;29(1):112–116.

Diette GB, White P Jr, Terry P, Jenckes M, Rosenthal D, Rubin HR. Utility of on-site cytopathology assessment for bronchoscopic evaluation of lung masses and adenopathy. *Chest.* 2000;117(4):1186–1190.

Ernst A, Feller-Kopman D, Herth FJ. Endobronchial ultrasound in the diagnosis and staging of lung cancer and other thoracic tumors. *Semin Thorac Cardiovasc Surg.* 2007;19(3):201–205.

Garpestad E, Goldberg SN, Herth F, Garland R, LoCicero J, Thurer R, Ernst A. CT fluoroscopy guidance for transbronchial needle aspiration: an experience in 35 patients. *Chest*. 2001;119(2):329–332.

Goldberg SN, Raptopoulos V, Boiselle PM, Edinburgh KJ, Ernst A. Mediastinal lymphadenopathy: diagnostic yield of transbronchial mediastinal lymph node biopsy with CT fluoroscopic guidance – initial experience. *Radiology*. 2000;216(3):764–767.

Haponik EF, Shure D. Underutilization of transbronchial needle aspiration: experiences of current pulmonary fellows. *Chest*. 1997;112(1):251–253.

Harrow EM, Abi-Saleh W, Blum J, Harkin T, Gasparini S, Addrizzo-Harris DJ, Arroliga AC, Wight G, Mehta AC. The utility of transbronchial needle aspiration in the staging of bronchogenic carcinoma. *Am J Respir Crit Care Med*. 2000;161(2 Pt 1):601–607.

Herth F, Becker HD, Ernst A. Conventional vs endo-bronchial ultrasound-guided transbronchial needle aspiration: a randomized trial. *Chest*. 2004;125(1):322–325.

Herth FJ, Becker HD, Ernst A. Ultrasound-guided trans-bronchial needle aspiration: an experience in 242 patients. *Chest*. 2003;123(2):604–607.

Herth FJ, Eberhardt R, Vilmann P, Krasnik M, Ernst A. Real-time, endobronchial ultrasound-guided, trans-bronchial needle aspiration: a new method for sampling mediastinal lymph nodes. *Thorax*. 2006;61(9):795–798. Epub 2006 May 31.

Herth FJF, Ernst A, Eberhardt R, Vilmann P, Diene-mann H, Krasnik M. Endobronchial ultrasound-guided transbronchial needle aspiration of lymph nodes in the radiologically normal mediastinum. *Eur Respir J*. 2006;28(5):910–914.

Holty JE, Kuschner WG, Gould MK. Accuracy of trans-bronchial needle aspiration for mediastinal staging of non-small cell lung cancer: a meta-analysis. *Thorax*. 2005;60(11):949–955.

Hsu LH, Liu CC, Ko JS. Education and experience improve the performance of transbronchial needle aspiration: a learning curve at a cancer center. *Chest*. 2004;125(2):532–540.

Kennedy MP, Jimenez CA, Bruzzi JF, Mhatre AD, Lei X, Giles FJ, Fanning T, Morice RC, Eapen GA. Endo-bronchial ultrasound guided transbronchial needle aspiration in the diagnosis of lymphoma. *Thorax*. 2008;63(4):360–365.

Oho K, Kato H, Ogawa I, Hayashi N, Hayata Y. A new needle for transfiberoptic bronchoscopic use. *Chest*. 1979;76(4):492.

Patel NM, Pohlman A, Husain A, Noth I, Hall JB, Kress JP. Conventional transbronchial needle aspiration decreases the rate of surgical sampling of intra-thoracic lymphadenopathy. *Chest*. 2007;131(3):773–778.

Schenk DA, Chambers SL, Derdak S, Komadina KH, Pickard JS, Strollo PJ, Lewis RE, Patefield AJ, Hen-derson JH. Comparison of the Wang 19-gauge and 22-gauge needles in the mediastinal staging of lung cancer. *Am Rev Respir Dis*. 1993;147(5):1251–1258.

Shure D, Fedullo PF. Transbronchial needle aspiration of peripheral masses. *Am Rev Respir Dis*. 1983;128(6):1090–1092.

Silvestri GA, Gould MK, Margolis ML, Tanoue LT, McCrory D, Toloza E, Detterbeck F. Noninvasive stag-ing of non-small cell lung cancer: ACCP evidenced-based clinical practice guidelines (2nd ed.). *Chest*. 2007;132(3 Suppl):178S–201S.

Vincent BD, El-Bayoumi E, Hoffman B, Doelken P, DeRosimo J, Reed C, Silvestri GA. Real-time endo-bronchial ultrasound-guided transbronchial lymph node aspiration. *Ann Thorac Surg*. 2008;85(1):224–230.

Wang KP. Staging of bronchogenic carcinoma by bron-choscopy. *Chest*. 1994;106(2):588–593.

Wang KP, Terry P, Marsh B. Bronchoscopic needle aspi-ration biopsy of paratracheal tumors. *Am Rev Respir Dis*. 1978;118(1):17–21.

Yasufuku K, Chiyo M, Sekine Y, Chhajed PN, Shibuya K, Iizasa T, Fujisawa T. Real-time endobronchial ultrasound-guided transbronchial needle aspiration of mediastinal and hilar lymph nodes. *Chest*. 2004;126(1):122–128.

12

BRONCHOSCOPY IN THE INTENSIVE CARE UNIT

Jed A. Gorden

In the future, as at present, the internist will tap and look and listen on the outside of the chest . . . ; the roentgenologist will continue to look through the patient; but in a continually increasing proportion of cases, the surgeon, the internist and the roentgenologist will ask the bronchoscopist to look inside the patient. – Chevalier Jackson, MD 1928

INTRODUCTION

Pulmonologists and surgeons are frequently called on to perform bronchoscopy on critically ill patients in the intensive care unit (ICU). The ease, safety, and portability of bronchoscopy make it one of the most commonly requested invasive procedures in the ICU setting. Flexible bronchoscopy (first fiber optic and now video) was introduced by Dr. Ikeda of Japan in the late 1960s and became more widely available in the mid to late 1970s. Now, with advances in technology allowing for greater portability, bronchoscopy has become ubiquitous in the modern hospital.

The ease of availability of bronchoscopy to intensivists has broadened the pulmonary diagnostic and therapeutic capabilities in critically ill patients, but like many technologies it also raises certain challenges in its appropriate application. Technology is not a substitute for good clinical judgment; operators must assess patient safety and perform procedures with attention to patient comfort and knowledge of potential complications and a management plan for complications including respiratory failure, pneumothorax, and so on.

In this chapter, I hope to outline the most common consultations and appropriate uses for bronchoscopy in the ICU. The overwhelming number of indications will be for diagnostic questions, although some therapeutic indications exist. Common indications for bronchoscopy in the ICU are listed in Table 12.1: The three most common requests are therapeutic aspiration of secretions, diagnosis of ventilator-associated pneumonia (VAP), and identification of the source of hemoptysis.

ROUTE OF BRONCHOSCOPY IN THE ICU

Bronchoscopy performed in the ICU on critically ill patients is safe, but an appropriate risk–benefit analysis is always necessary. Bronchoscopy can be performed on both intubated and extubated patients, but when bronchoscopy is performed on extubated patients, stability of oxygenation and ventilation must be assessed and the risk of respiratory failure from sedation, medications, or the procedure itself must be determined.

Bronchoscopy in the Extubated Patient
Bronchoscopy on the extubated patient can be performed either via the oral route using a bite block or transnasally. The patient must have oxygen requirements that can be managed by reasonable supplementation and cannot have impending respiratory failure or requirements for noninvasive ventilation like continuous positive airway pressure (CPAP) or bilevel positive airway pressure (BIPAP). The patient should have a mental status that permits the

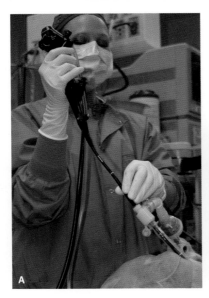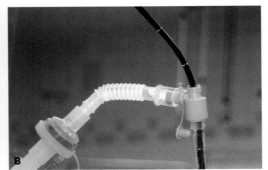

FIGURE 12.1. **(A)** Bronchoscopy performed through an ETT. **(B)** An adapter is attached to the ETT to permit continuous mechanical ventilation and simultaneous bronchoscopic access to the airway.

use of sedation and analgesia. The bronchoscopist, when performing bronchoscopy on an extubated ICU patient, must be knowledgeable about intubation and skilled in intubation either by direct laryngoscopy or over a bronchoscope, in case of respiratory failure. Contraindications to flexible bronchoscopy without intubation include (1) respiratory rate > 30 bpm, (2) clinical use of accessory muscles signifying impending respiratory failure, (3) partial pressure of oxygen in arterial blood (PaO$_2$) < 70 mm Hg or peripheral capillary oxygen saturation (SaO$_2$) < 90% with supplemental oxygen, (4) a requirement for minimally invasive BIPAP/CPAP ventilation, and (5) significantly altered mental status.

Bronchoscopy in the Intubated Patient

Performing bronchoscopy through an endotracheal tube (ETT) in the ICU is a common procedure. The ETT should be placed prior to the procedure if the patient's respiratory status is felt to be fragile and the information from bronchoscopy is critical to patient care. The inner

diameters of ETTs in common use in adults are 7.0 mm, 7.5 mm, and 8.0 mm. The outer diameter of the common diagnostic bronchoscope is approximately 5 mm. The bronchoscope must easily pass through the inner lumen of the ETT and permit exhaled gas to escape to prevent air trapping; to achieve this, an 8.0-mm ETT is most desirable, and a 7.5-mm ETT can be considered. If the patient has a smaller diameter ETT the intensivist should consider changing the ETT to a larger diameter. If the airway does not permit a larger ETT because of stenosis or another cause, consider using a pediatric or smaller diameter bronchoscope. Remember that a smaller bronchoscope will have a smaller working channel and considerably less suctioning capability, limiting visibility and decreasing suctioning of secretions and specimen acquisition.

When performing bronchoscopy on the mechanically ventilated patient, an adapter is required on the end of the ETT to permit access to the airway while ensuring that tidal volume and positive end-expiratory pressure are maintained during the procedure (Figure 12.1).

Sedation

When bronchoscopy is performed on either the intubated or extubated patient in the ICU, sedation is required. Typical sedation involves the use of an analgesic and a sedative. The most common combination is opiates and benzodiazepines, but sedation can be individualized to your specific ICU protocol. Topical sedation for both the intubated and extubated patient cannot be overlooked. In the extubated patient, topical anesthesia in the posterior pharynx and airway limits the gag reflex. In the intubated patient, topical anesthesia down the ETT or tracheostomy tube minimizes airway cough. Lidocaine 1%–2%, 2 cc in a 5-cc syringe with 3 cc of air, allows for good delivery of drug and anesthetizes the airway and decreases cough. When bronchoscopy is to be performed via the nasal route, the nares must be adequately anesthetized. For ICU bronchoscopy, routine neuromuscular blockade is not required.

In general, patients undergoing bronchoscopy in the ICU should have had no oral or tube feed intake for 6 hours prior to the procedure. If the patient is taking spontaneous meals they should be held, and if the patient is receiving tube feeds these also should be held for 6 hours prior to the procedure. The patient can be maintained with intravenous hydration during this period.

SAFETY OF BRONCHOSCOPY IN THE CRITICALLY ILL

Flexible bronchoscopy and sample acquisition from the airways that it affords is a valuable tool of the critical care physician. The question of safety of bronchoscopy in the critically ill has been extensively evaluated in the literature.

Patients admitted to the critical care setting suffer from a variety of organ system failures, some with causes readily diagnosed and others more illusive. A common thread in many ICU patients is the diagnostic dilemma posed by the abnormal chest x-ray and the concern for infection, bleeding or airway obstruction. The severity of illness (respiratory failure, hemodynamic compromise, or other critical organ system dysfunction) should not be considered a barrier to bronchoscopy and obtaining valuable data that could impact patient management.

Diagnostic bronchoscopy with bronchoalveolar lavage (BAL) or protected specimen brush (PSB) is safe even in patients who meet clinical criteria for adult respiratory distress syndrome, defined as PaO_2/fraction of inspired oxygen (FiO_2) ≤ 200 diffuse bilateral parenchymal infiltrates on x-ray, and no evidence of volume overload. In this type of patient, you should be able to perform bronchoscopy with BAL or brushing with little or no clinically significant change in the patient's mean PaO_2/FiO_2 ratio, mean arterial pressure, or heart rate when comparing preprocedure values with 1-hour postprocedure vitals. What you may expect in some patients is a transient drop in SaO_2 during installation of lavage fluid, but patients should recover in about 15 minutes of procedure without any long-term sequelae from the transient desaturation. Changes in oxygen saturations or other vital signs during the procedure rarely if ever are a cause to abort the procedure prematurely.

Another large patient population in the ICU is hemodynamically unstable patients who often require ionotropic and/or vasoactive support. In this patient population, bronchoscopy is also safe, including the use of lavage fluid and brush-collected specimens. No prophylactic increases in vasoactive support are required, nor are any clinically significant hemodynamic changes expected (3).

In clinical settings where bronchoscopy and BAL have been used in critically ill patients, safety was maintained despite the installation of 100–200 cc of 0.9% saline for lavage. No temperature adjustments of lavage fluid or changes in volume are required. One of the advantages of serial installations of lavage fluid is to not just sample the airway but to create a column of fluid to sample the alveolar bed.

Table 12.1. *Indications for bronchoscopy in the ICU*

Diagnostic	Therapeutic
Secretion/atelectasis management	Hemoptysis
Fever/ventilator-associated pneumonia	Foreign body removal
Hemoptysis	Difficult intubations
Failed extubation	Percutaneous tracheostomy guidance
Undiagnosed x-ray change	
Central airway obstruction	

Table 12.2. *Contraindications to bronchoscopy in the ICU*

Patient PaO_2 <60–80 mm Hg on 100% FiO_2
Acute ischemic heart disease (MI) or unstable angina
Hypotension with systemic blood pressure <90 mm Hg
Critical cardiac dysrhythmias
Known increased intracranial pressures

Note: MI, myocardial infarction.

The two most common and most studied bronchoscopic procedures in critically ill patients are BAL and PSB, both very safe. A less commonly used and more controversial procedure in the ICU is the transbronchial biopsy. The risks of performing transbronchial biopsy in all patients are pneumothorax and bleeding. The risk of inducing a pneumothorax is not necessarily increased in mechanically ventilated patients, but the consequences (including tension pneumothorax caused by positive pressure ventilation) are greater. The use of uniplanar fluoroscopy does not minimize the risk of pneumothorax; only experience and good technique lower the risk. The clinician must perform a careful risk–benefit analysis on the value of a transbronchial biopsy specimen before performing one. Common ICU problems (including coagulopathy and platelet dysfunction, as well as therapeutic anticoagulation with warfarin or heparin) are absolute contraindications to the use of transbronchial biopsy.

Bronchoscopy is considered safe in critically ill patients with both respiratory failure and hemodynamic impairment as long as simple principles are followed. To safely perform bronchoscopy in critically ill patients, a knowledgeable team is required. Staffing should include a respiratory therapist at the bedside as well as a nurse present to assist with sedation and monitoring. An assistant is required to assist with specimen acquisition. Indications and contraindications as well as a safety checklist for flexible bronchoscopy in the ICU are outlined in Tables 12.1, 12.2 and 12.3. Bronchoscopy should be avoided in the following clinical circumstances: (1) PaO_2 < 60–80 mm Hg on 100% FiO_2, (2) acute ischemic heart disease or unstable angina, (3) hypotension with systolic blood pressure, (4) critical cardiac dysrhythmias, and/or (5) known increased intracranial pressure.

To safely perform bronchoscopy on critically ill patients, the following are required: (1) continuous oxygen saturation monitoring; (2) monitoring of hemodynamics every 2–5 minutes; (3) in ventilated patients, the FiO_2 increased to 100% 5–15 minutes prior to the procedure; and (4) monitoring for loss of minute ventilation and pressure-limited volume loss caused by the presence of the bronchoscope in the airway increasing peak airway pressures.

Table 12.3. *Bronchoscopy safety checklist*

Continuous oxygen saturation monitoring
Hemodynamic monitoring cycled every 2–5 minutes
Continuous cardiac rate and rhythm monitoring
Ventilated patients increase FiO_2 to 100% 5–15 minutes prior to procedure
Nursing support for sedation and monitoring
Respiratory therapy support for ventilator management monitoring of minute ventilation and pressure-limited volume loss
Technical support to assist with procedure, lavage, etc.

BRONCHOSCOPY IN FEBRILE NEUTROPENIA

Febrile neutropenic patients are a specialty group of patients often admitted to the ICU setting. Febrile neutropenia is considered an oncologic emergency and is most commonly associated with the use of chemotherapy or hematopoietic stem cell transplantation. Febrile neutropenia alone carries a mortality rate of approximately 10%. When febrile neutropenia is accompanied by pulmonary infiltrates, the mortality rate can approach 40%. When respiratory failure requiring mechanical ventilation occurs in the setting of febrile neutropenia, the mortality rate can exceed 90%. The differential diagnosis for febrile neutropenia and pulmonary infiltrates can be broad, with infection (bacterial, fungal, or viral) being the most sinister. Other diagnoses include, but are not limited to, diffuse alveolar hemorrhage, radiation pneumonitis, drug-induced toxicity, or malignancy itself.

Early use of empiric antibiotic therapy is the standard of care for this patient population, but flexible bronchoscopy is both safe and commonly used to augment the diagnostic workup. Diagnostic yield of flexible bronchoscopy in the febrile neutropenic patient in multiple studies has been shown to be approximately 50%. In febrile neutropenic patients, the diagnostic yield of flexible bronchoscopy and BAL differs because of neutropenia. In patients who experience febrile neutropenia as a result of high-dose chemotherapy, the diagnostic yield of bronchoscopy and BAL is about 60%; if the cause of neutropenia is stem cell transplantation, the diagnostic yield is lower (35%–50% on average). This lower yield may reflect that other factors besides infection are at play in the bone marrow transplant population.

Bronchoscopy in the febrile neutropenic patient in the ICU is safe, with complications usually being minor and most always mirroring those of the general critically ill population. A unique clinical finding in this patient population (in addition to their critical illness) is

thrombocytopenia, either as a result of medications or underlying illness. Flexible bronchoscopy in the setting of thrombocytopenia is safe and is rarely associated with hemoptysis or alveolar hemorrhage or other bleeding complications. Bronchoscopy in thrombocytopenia can safely be performed via the oral or nasal route, as well as in the intubated patient. There is no absolute lower limit of platelet count to safely perform bronchoscopy with BAL, and routine platelet transfusions are not required.

Nearly all patients with febrile neutropenia are on empiric broad-spectrum antibiotics when the bronchoscopist is consulted to perform BAL. BAL results will produce a change in antimicrobial therapy in nearly a quarter to one half of cases. Viral and fungal diseases often account for most therapeutic changes. *Aspergillus* often represents the most common organism recovered, found in nearly 20% of samples. A nondiagnostic bronchoscopy with BAL is insufficient to discontinue antimicrobial therapy in this patient population. In cases of nondiagnostic BAL, a careful review of clinical circumstances beyond the scope of this review is warranted in consideration of alternative diagnostic procedures including surgical lung biopsy.

Transbronchial biopsy in the febrile neutropenic patient adds little to the diagnostic yield and is usually considered contraindicated in the setting of thrombocytopenia. PSBs, if used to collect mucoid secretions, are safe in thrombocytopenia, but if the brush is used to disrupt the mucosa for cellular collection, this should be considered contraindicated in the setting of thrombocytopenia.

In summary, flexible bronchoscopy in the setting of critical illness and febrile neutropenia is safe in the presence or absence of thrombocytopenia. The diagnostic yield is approximately 50%. Accurate microbiologic data are critical to clinical decision making, and BAL results can alter therapy in a quarter to one half of these patients. Mortality of febrile neutropenic patients in respiratory failure requiring mechanical ventilation is high, but when a proven infectious diagnosis is made there is a significantly lower mortality.

THERAPEUTIC ASPIRATION OF SECRETIONS

One of the most common consultations for bronchoscopy in the ICU is the management of retained secretions and atelectasis. In published series from the Mayo Clinic ICU from 1985 through 1988, clearance of retained secretions accounted for 50% of ICU bronchoscopies, and in a series from the University of California Davis from 1979 through 1980, 63% of bronchoscopies were performed for this purpose. The use of bronchoscopy for retained secretions and atelectasis is the subject of strong convictions and few data. There is little doubt that bronchoscopy for therapeutic removal of secretions and aggressive pulmonary toilet is safe, but its efficacy and impact on clinical outcomes remains unresolved. When therapeutic bronchoscopy has been compared with aggressive pulmonary toilet there has been little difference in outcomes, and when air bronchograms are present, Figure 12.2, both strategies are equally bad at resolving atelectasis.

Bronchoscopy and BAL should not be considered first-line therapy for routine pulmonary toilet and secretion clearance in the ICU. Bron-

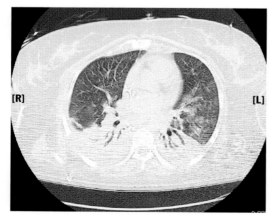

FIGURE 12.2. CT scan of the chest showing bilateral posterior air bronchograms.

choscopy should be considered in cases of acute lobar collapse, particularly with alterations in oxygenation status if routine suctioning fails. In cases of lobar atelectasis with or without air bronchograms, bronchoscopy should be considered if endobronchial obstruction either from foreign body or tumor is suspected.

VENTILATOR-ASSOCIATED PNEUMONIA

Ventilator-associated pneumonia (VAP) is a common and serious problem facing critically ill patients on mechanical ventilation. It is estimated that 8%–28% of intubated patients requiring mechanical ventilation will develop a VAP. Mortality associated with VAP is high (between 24% and 50%). Given the severe consequences associated with VAP, it is critical that a timely and accurate diagnosis is made. Bronchoscopy with BAL is an excellent tool for making the diagnosis of VAP. Directed specimens from focal areas suspicious on chest x-ray allow physicians to develop a powerful and accurate strategy for antibiotic use superior to most routine clinical means. The use of quantitative cultures obtained by BAL or PSB, although not without controversy, has been associated with a decreased mortality from VAP, less organ dysfunction, and less antibiotic use in a randomized controlled trial. Colonization versus true infection is an important issue that can be addressed by the use of directed quantitative cultures and is the critical issue in the debate over the use of an invasive versus noninvasive sampling strategy.

In many critically ill patients, bilateral infiltrates are present, thus complicating decision making for directed quantitative BAL. Unilateral acquisition of a specimen could lead to an erroneous treatment plan. When new bilateral suspicious infiltrates are present on chest x-ray, a bilateral directed bronchoscopic lavage should be performed.

Bronchoscopy should not delay antimicrobial therapy, particularly in ICU settings where 24-hour bronchoscopy services are not available.

When available, quantitative cultures obtained by bronchoscopy help to tailor antibiotic therapy even if the overall effects of bronchoscopy and BAL on VAP and mortality remain controversial. In mechanically ventilated patients, VAP should be suspected and bronchoscopy initiated when (1) a patient has been on mechanical ventilation for >48 hours with new or persistent infiltrates on chest x-ray and (2) one of the following: purulent secretions, febrile temperature >38.3°C, and leukocytosis. When bilateral infiltrates are present, consider the use of bilateral quantitative BAL.

HEMOPTYSIS

The goals in managing massive hemoptysis are securing of the airway, identification of the bleeding source, isolation of the bleeding area to prevent soiling of the unaffected lung, and cessation of bleeding. No consensus definition exists for massive hemoptysis; the literature often quotes 100–600 cc/24 h, but it is most important to understand that problems come not from blood loss but impairment in gas exchange. Four hundred milliliters of blood in the alveolar space can significantly impair gas exchange with only a minor perturbation in vital signs. Bronchoscopy and radiology imaging are potent tools in identifying the cause and location of hemoptysis. Bronchoscopy allows for direct examination of the central airways for tumors or other bleeding diathesis as well as examination of segmental orifices to reveal the potential regional source of bleeding or, at a minimum, lateralize the source of bleeding to the left or right lung. Timing is crucial in localizing bleeding in cases of hemoptysis. When bronchoscopy is performed early either during active bleeding or shortly thereafter, bleeding can be localized in 75%–85% of cases. When bronchoscopy is delayed beyond the immediate bleeding period, localization falls to 25%–50%.

Computed tomography (CT) imaging is far superior to conventional chest x-ray and greatly helps the bronchoscopist by creating a potential road map of airway and parenchymal abnormalities. The intensivist must take into account the patient's stability when considering the role of medical imaging because it would be inappropriate to transfer an unstable patient to radiology.

Localization of non-life-threatening hemoptysis is best done using the flexible bronchoscope. It is rapidly available, does not require general anesthesia, can be used at the bedside, and allows for the most thorough airway survey. This rapid diagnostic survey helps with therapeutic planning. Diagnostic bronchoscopy should be done early, within 24 hours of bleeding, to maximize the chances of localizing or, at a minimum, lateralizing the bleeding source. The primary limitations of flexible bronchoscopy are diminished visibility (even in the presence of small volumes of blood) and low suction capability. In the presence of active bleeding, it may be difficult for the flexible bronchoscope to adequately obtain and maintain a clear airway, limiting both the goal of airway control and the goal of bleeding localization.

When the bleeding source has been localized, good communication is required between the bronchoscopist and his or her therapeutic colleagues in interventional pulmonology, thoracic surgery, or interventional radiology. A number of interventional options (beyond the scope of this review) are available for central airway bleeding lesions, including heat energy sources, APC, laser, and cautery. If the source of bleeding has been localized beyond the central airways, good anatomical communication with interventional radiology colleagues is necessary for potential embolization procedures; for patients with known malignancy despite localized control, consultation with radiation oncology provides another therapeutic option.

If bleeding is extensive, the use of endobronchial tamponade using endobronchial blockers is an important temporizing tool while awaiting more definitive therapy. Endobronchial blockers can be placed under direct vision using flexible bronchoscopy (Figure 12.3). After the

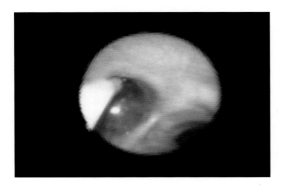

FIGURE 12.3. Inflated bronchial blocker occluding a bronchial orifice.

blocker is inflated, it should be deflated and the airway inspected at least every 24 hours.

In extreme life-threatening cases, selective intubation of either the right or left main stem bronchi is required to prevent soiling the unaffected lung. This is best and most rapidly achieved by placing the endotracheal tube over the bronchoscope, advancing the bronchoscope into the nonbleeding lung and advancing the endotracheal tube into the selected main stem airway. Using the bronchoscope as a guide wire, inflate the balloon on the endotracheal tube to prevent soiling.

A practical approach to massive hemoptysis is outlined in Figure 12.4, but the principles include (1) early patient stabilization with attention to the airway and breathing and the potential need for intubation, (2) early localization

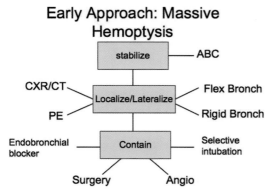

FIGURE 12.4. **Management algorithm for massive hemoptysis**. ABC, airway, breathing and circulation; CXR, chest x-ray; PE, physical exam.

of bleeding with bronchoscopy and possible CT imaging, and finally (3) containment of bleeding with localized therapy or interventional radiology embolization.

Massive hemoptysis requires a true multidisciplinary approach, and good early communication between intensivists and interventionalists from many disciplines including interventional pulmonology, thoracic surgery, interventional radiology, and radiation oncology is required.

REMOVAL OF FOREIGN BODY

In March of 1897, Professor Killian was presented with a 63-year-old farmer with profound dyspnea, cough, and hemoptysis. Killian, using the Kirstein laryngoscope, identified an object in the right main stem bronchus. Using cocaine anesthesia and the Mickulicz–Rosenheim esophagoscope, Killian deployed graspers through the lumen of the scope to secure what turned out to be a pork bone fragment. The 8-mm diameter of the esophagoscope forced the en masse removal of the object and the scope, and thus the first documented bronchoscopic procedure was performed for a foreign body extraction.

Aspiration of a foreign body can lead to critical airway obstruction and respiratory distress or obstruction at the segmental level resulting in lobar collapse or postobstructive pneumonia (Figure 12.5). The ease of access to the airways with bronchoscopy has had a dramatic impact on the subacute and chronic sequelae associated with airway foreign bodies, namely respiratory distress, obstructive pneumonia, and lung abscess, and has significantly lowered the mortality associated with foreign body aspiration. The nature of aspirated foreign bodies has certain geographic and cultural variability. The most cited foreign body aspirations are vegetable matter, peanuts, or bones. Not all foreign bodies are aspirated in the outpatient setting. Hospital appliances, particularly tracheal appliances including tracheal buttons, can find their way into the airway. The most common age groups for foreign body aspiration are children under

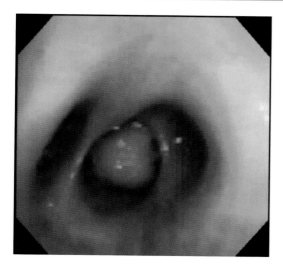

FIGURE 12.5. Airway obstruction with aspirated vegetable matter.

the age of 3 and adults in the sixth and seventh decades of life. The predominance of aspirated foreign bodies occurs in children.

Flexible bronchoscopy is a powerful tool in the removal of aspirated foreign bodies; its safety and portability profile make it an excellent ICU bedside tool for this purpose. In one published series, flexible bronchoscopy was successful in extracting a foreign body from the airway in 60% of cases. It is reasonable to initially attempt foreign body extraction with the flexible bronchoscope, with a high likelihood of success, but rigid bronchoscopy is a useful adjunct, and prompt conversion to rigid bronchoscopy may save the patient from multiple interventions.

It is generally thought that, when aspiration occurs, objects preferentially obstruct the right bronchial tree because of the anatomy and angle of entry into the right and left main stem bronchi off the trachea. In adults, the left main stem bronchus branches at a more obtuse angle relative to the midline trachea in contrast the right main stem bronchus, which maintains a more direct linear path with the trachea resulting in more frequent right main stem bronchial intubations as well as aspiration of foreign objects.

Factors that can impact aspiration risk include level of consciousness, age, and facial trauma. When these factors are present and are coupled with unexplained lobar collapse or unexplained wheezing, a diagnostic bronchoscopy should be considered to rule out an aspirated foreign body.

BRONCHOSCOPY IN TRAUMA

Airway trauma can occur as a result of external blunt force injuries or internal insults like the ETT stilet. Airway injuries can be readily identified by bedside bronchoscopy. Common traumatic injuries associated with tracheal or bronchial disruption include pneumomediastinum post blunt trauma to the chest, persistent pneumothorax despite adequate chest tube evacuation in the setting of thoracic trauma, and fracture of one or more of the first three ribs. These signs of airway injury may be overlooked in critically ill patients suffering from blunt force traumatic injury to the chest; therefore, with close consultation with the surgeon diagnostic bronchoscopy should be considered in these patients after the initial trauma resuscitation is complete.

In cases of persistent pneumomediastinum, without other explanation, airway injury can be suspected, including airway injury sustained as a result of intubation with a stilet. Typically this results in injury to the posterior membranous trachea or the right main stem bronchus if the ETT is advanced too far. Again, this can be readily diagnosed by flexible bronchoscopy but may require deflation of the balloon on the ETT and gentle withdrawal of the tube if the ETT has been advanced over the injury site.

Inhalation injury (either steam or caustic substances) warrants an airway inspection to assess for airway sloughing and web stenosis formation. It can also be used to assess for laryngeal swelling and the need for securing a stable airway.

FAILED EXTUBATION

Failure to be able to liberate a patient from mechanical ventilation is a common problem in the ICU and most often reflects persistent critical illness and respiratory failure. In certain circumstances, failure to extubate reflects a mechanical problem that increases the work of breathing. Specific mechanical problems that can be readily diagnosed by bronchoscopy are (1) increased airway granulation tissue resulting in airway obstruction, (2) tracheal stenosis, and (3) tracheal bronchial malacia. These clinical conditions are easily diagnosed by bedside bronchoscopy.

ICU SPECIAL CIRCUMSTANCES

The bronchoscope should always be considered part of the difficult intubation armamentarium. In the case of a difficult airway, intubation can be facilitated by placing the ETT over the bronchoscope, using the bronchoscopic optics to find the cords and pass into the trachea, then advancing the ETT over the bronchoscope into the airway. This maneuver is easiest when one is using a 7.5- or 8.0-mm ETT, which allows for the use of a regular diagnostic bronchoscope. The larger the diameter of the scope, the easier it is to maneuver and to aspirate secretions to improve visibility. If a smaller ETT is required because of airway compromise, a smaller bronchoscope is required. This technique is useful in patients who cannot extend their neck because of either trauma or other causes of instability that contraindicate direct laryngoscopy.

Increasingly tracheostomy tubes in ICUs are being placed at the bedsides of patients who require prolonged mechanical ventilation. Bronchoscopy is required to ensure midline placement and safe passage of the airway dilator so as to minimize the risk of injury to the posterior membrane of the trachea.

Inspection of central airway obstruction is best performed by flexible bronchoscopy after the patient's airway has been stabilized. Direct visual inspection of the airway allows for greater planning of therapeutic procedures including appropriate stent sizing and airway debridement. Although the definitive management of central airway obstruction is best performed in the operating room with rigid bronchoscopy, a preprocedure inspection with flexible bronchoscopy is critical to planning.

SUMMARY

Bronchoscopy is a tool that is now widely available in hospitals. The combined ability of direct visualization and sample acquisition makes it extremely useful in the diagnosis of chest diseases. Incorporating this potent tool in the critical care setting is becoming more and more regular. In critically ill patients, bronchoscopy is a safe tool, when appropriately applied, and it extends our diagnostic capabilities. In certain circumstances, bronchoscopy improves safety in fragile, critically ill patients. The use of bronchoscopy in the ICU requires good clinical judgment backed by appropriate training and a skilled supporting team.

SUGGESTED READINGS

Chastre J, Fagon JY. Ventilator-associated pneumonia. *Am J Respir Crit Care Med.* 2002;165:867–903.

Debeljaak A, Sorli J, Music E, Kecelj P. Bronchoscopic removal of foreign bodies in adults: experience with 62 patients from 1974–1998. *Eur Respir J.* 1999;14(4):792–795.

Fagon JY, Chastre J, Wolff M, et al. Invasive and noninvasive strategies for management of suspected ventilator-associated pneumonia. *Ann Intern Med.* 2000;132:621–630.

Gong H, Salvatierra C. Clinical efficacy of early and delayed fiberoptic bronchoscopy in patients with hemoptysis. *Am Rev Respir Dis.* 1981;124:221–225.

Gruson D, Hilbert G, Valentino R, et al. Utility of fiberoptic bronchoscopy in neutropenic patients admitted to the intensive care unit with pulmonary infiltrates. *Crit Care Med.* 2000;28:2224–2230.

Hertz MI, Woodward ME, Gross CR, Swart M, Marcy TW, Bitterman PB. Safety of bronchoalveolar lavage in the critically ill, mechanically ventilated patient. *Crit Care Med.* 1991;19(12):1526–1532.

Jackson SR, Ernst NE, Mueller EW, Butler KL. Utility of bronchoalveolar lavage for the diagnosis of ventilator-associated pneumonia in critically ill surgical patients. *Am J Surg.* 2008;195:159–163.

Kelly SM, Marsh BR. Airway foreign bodies. *Chest Surg Clin N Am.* 1996;6(2):253–276.

Kreider ME, Lipson D. Bronchoscopy for atelectasis in the ICU: a case report and review of the literature. *Chest.* 2003;124:344–350.

Lan RS. Non-asphyxiating tracheobronchial foreign bodies in adults. *Eur Respir J.* 1994;7(3):510–514.

Marini JJ, Pierson DJ, Hudson LD. Acute lobar atelectasis: a prospective comparison of fiberoptic bronchoscopy and respiratory therapy. *Am Rev Respir Dis.* 1979;119:971–978.

Papazian L, Colt HG, Scemama F, Martin C, Gouin F. Effects of consecutive protected specimen brushing and bronchoalveolar lavage on gas exchange and hemodynamics in ventilated patients. *Chest.* 1993;104:1548–1552.

Pursel SE, Lindskog GE. Hemoptysis: a clinical evaluation of 105 patients examined consecutively on a thoracic surgical service. *Am Rev Respir Dis.* 1961;84:329–336.

Rafanan AL, Mehta AC. Adult airway foreign body removal. What's new? *Clin Chest Med.* 2001;22(2):319–330.

Saw EC, Gottlieb LS, Yokoyama T, Lee BC. Flexible fiberoptic bronchoscopy and endobronchial tamponade in the management of massive hemoptysis. *Chest.* 1976;70:589–591.

Steinberg KP, Mitchell DR, Maunder RJ, Milberg JA, Whitcomb ME. Safety of bronchoalveolar lavage in patients with adult respiratory distress syndrome. *Am Rev Respir Dis.* 1993;148:556–561.

Zollner F. Gustav Killian, father of bronchoscopy. *Arch Otolaryngol.* 1965;82:656–659.

13

BRONCHOSCOPY IN THE LUNG TRANSPLANT PATIENT

Anne L. Fuhlbrigge

INTRODUCTION

Lung transplantation has rapidly evolved since the first operation in the early 1960s and has become an established treatment for a variety of patients with end-stage lung disease. Bronchoscopy is an essential tool in the diagnosis and management of lung transplant recipients. In this chapter we will outline four areas in which bronchoscopy plays a critical role in the care of patients undergoing lung transplantation: (1) evaluation of potential lung donors, (2) surveillance for acute rejection, (3) evaluation and treatment among lung transplant recipients presenting with new symptoms or deteriorating respiratory function, and (4) visualization of the anastomosis and management of airway complications.

THE ROLE OF BRONCHOSCOPY IN THE ASSESSMENT OF POTENTIAL LUNG DONORS

Flexible bronchoscopy is an essential part of the evaluation of all potential lung donors. Bronchoscopy can assess for evidence of lung injury, inflammation, aspiration, and infection. If bronchoscopy shows no anatomic abnormality, endobronchial lesions, or secretions, acceptance of the organ for donation is appropriate. However, only about one third of persons meeting criteria

for brain death, and being considered for donation, will have a normal bronchoscopy. A normal bronchoscopy is not a requirement for accepting a potential lung donor; the findings on flexible bronchoscopy can help select donors acceptable for donation and donors that should be rejected.

Detailed Inspection of the Anatomy

An important finding during bronchoscopy is the presence of anatomic variations that influence the operative procedure and potential use of the organ. As an example, the author has encountered a potential donor in which the orifice for the right upper lobe (RUL) was located very proximally in relation to the carina, making anastomosis difficult without sacrificing the RUL during the procedure. Decisions regarding specific anatomic variants and how they might impact the use of a potential donor should be routinely discussed with the accepting transplant surgeon.

Obtaining Microbiologic Samples

Aspiration and pneumonia are common in potential donors, yet the presence of mucopurulent secretions among donors without clear evidence of pneumonia and a clear chest x-ray is common. Bronchoscopy can guide the selection of organs. If extensive endobronchial inflammation is seen or if extensive secretions emanate from the distal segments that do not readily clear, the donor may have suffered an aspiration event

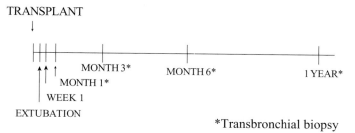

TRANSPLANT

MONTH 3*
MONTH 1*
WEEK 1
EXTUBATION

MONTH 6*

1 YEAR*

*Transbronchial biopsy

FIGURE 13.1. Sample schedule for routine surveillance bronchoscopy at a single lung transplant center. Surveillance bronchoscopy to assess anastomotic healing and to aid in pulmonary clearance is performed prior to extubation and at 1 week post-transplant. Routine surveillance bronchoscopy with transbronchial biopsy is performed at 1, 3, 6, and 12 months post-transplant.

and may be developing an infection that precludes accepting the lung for donation, despite a clear chest x-ray. Alternatively, if the endobronchial mucosa is normal in appearance and the secretions are easily suctioned clear without recurrent welling up during the examination, the potential donor lungs are likely appropriate for use. In this situation, bronchoscopy can also be used to obtain specimens to facilitate targeted antimicrobial therapy in the recipient during the immediate postoperative period. There is debate regarding the importance of a positive Gram stain in the selection of donors for transplantation, but prior studies have shown no correlation between a positive donor Gram stain and subsequent postoperative pneumonia in the recipient.

SURVEILLANCE BRONCHOSCOPY

Close surveillance of the allograft is the key to a successful transplant outcome. In many transplant centers, routine surveillance bronchoscopy at predetermined time intervals for the evaluation of acute rejection is a central component of this surveillance (Figure 13.1).

Recent surveys of transplant programs across the United States and internationally documented that more than 50% of programs perform surveillance procedures. Transbronchial biopsy is the gold standard for the diagnosis of acute rejection, with sensitivities in the range of 93% reported for acute rejection; however,

studies have shown a false-negative rate of between 15% and 28%. Variation in yield may be related to technique as published reports have varied in their sampling methods (from 3 pieces in one lobe to 17 pieces from both lungs). At most centers in the United States, a biopsy is taken from only one lung to avoid the risk of bilateral pneumothoraces. A decision regarding the number of biopsies is a balance is between obtaining enough biopsies to achieve an adequate diagnostic yield and avoiding a high risk of complications. The consensus recommendation is that a specimen containing five pieces of alveolated lung parenchyma, each with a minimum of 100 alveoli and bronchioles, is necessary to minimize the risk of sampling error and false-negative results and to optimize yield.

Lung transplant recipients are at highest risk of acute rejection in the first 6–12 months following lung transplant. However, chronic rejection is rarely seen before 6 months. In addition, the presence of chronic rejection in biopsies does not correlate well with functional status, and the diagnostic yield from flexible bronchoscopy in chronic rejection is much lower than that in acute rejection. Therefore, lung transplant centers do not perform surveillance bronchoscopy with transbronchial lung biopsy (TBBx) after the first year to monitor for the development of chronic rejection. The diagnosis and staging of chronic lung allograft dysfunction, bronchiolitis obliterans syndrome (BOS), is based on clinical criteria (forced expiratory volume in 1 second

[FEV$_1$]) and is defined as graft deterioration caused by progressive airway disease for which there is no evidence of another superimposed process. Bronchoscopy does play an important role in excluding other treatable causes of graft dysfunction but cannot routinely confirm the diagnosis of chronic rejection.

The use of routine surveillance transbronchial biopsies remains an area of debate among clinicians and was the focus of a recent pro–con debate at the international meeting of the American Thoracic Society. Proponents underscore the frequency of unexpected findings during surveillance bronchoscopy; up to one quarter to one third of specimens during the first year can influence management. This is confirmed by a report from a program that performed surveillance bronchoscopy among clinically healthy lung transplant recipients and found significant abnormalities in a large proportion of patients; 39% had some degree of acute rejection, 14% had evidence of cytomegalovirus, 18% had nonspecific findings, with only 24% being read as normal. Importantly, it has been demonstrated that asymptomatic mild acute rejection, when left untreated, can progress to symptomatic higher grade rejection. In addition, patients who experience multiple low-grade rejections in the first year of transplant may develop earlier onset chronic rejection, independent of whether they go on to develop higher grades of rejection, suggesting that these patients may warrant more aggressive immunosuppression. Finally, the importance of follow-up bronchoscopy after a documented episode of rejection is highlighted, demonstrating that persistent rejection is found in many cases that required further treatment.

In contrast, opponents of routine surveillance bronchoscopy with transbronchial biopsy highlight the lack of data showing a significant difference in long-term outcome among patients in whom surveillance bronchoscopy is performed, compared with patients in whom bronchoscopy is performed only when clinically indicated by symptoms or decrease in lung function. In addition, opponents highlight the costs of repeated

procedures and the associated risk of complications. No randomized controlled trials have examined this issue, and the available data to guide this decision come from retrospective, nonrandomized studies with their inherent limitations.

DIAGNOSTIC BRONCHOSCOPY FOR EVALUATION OF CLINICAL DETERIORATION

Diagnostic bronchoscopy can provide valuable information in lung transplant recipients when they present with new respiratory symptoms or a decline in functional status. Pulmonary infections in lung transplant patients can be difficult to diagnose. The presenting signs and symptoms are similar between infectious and noninfectious complications of transplantation. DeVito Dabbs and colleagues found no significant differences in the severity or type of symptoms between patients who were diagnosed with an infection versus those found to have rejection. Bronchoscopy with bronchoalveolar lavage (BAL) and TBBx play a critical role in differentiating these two entities, and interpretation of the biopsy should be made in light of the entire clinical, microbiologic, and radiographic picture. There are some reports highlighting the role of cell counts and differentials counts in the management of lung transplant recipients, but the routine use of this has not been adopted in all centers.

Infection represents a leading cause of death in the first year after transplant, with the rate of infection being higher among lung transplant patients compared with other solid organ transplant patients. The reasons for this increased risk of infection are several, but a primary reason is the required suppression of humoral and cell-mediated immunity by immunosuppressant therapy. The dosing of immunosuppressant medications is highest during the first year secondary to a higher risk of rejection during this same period. Therefore, the balance of competing risks, infection and rejection, is more difficult in the first year (Figure 13.2).

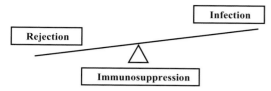

FIGURE 13.2. Illustration of the pivotal role immunosuppressive therapy plays in the balance between the risk of rejection and risk of infection among lung transplant recipients. This balance is particularly difficult in the first year post-transplant.

Other changes in the innate defense of lung transplant patients play a role in the increased risk of infection. In the immediate postoperative period, lung transplant recipients have a blunted cough reflex because of postoperative pain and the denervation of the lung that occurs. This contributes to poor clearance of respiratory secretions and the potential for microaspiration, which is aggravated in many patients by postoperative gastroparesis. In addition, poor lymphatic drainage, impaired mucociliary clearance secondary to ischemic injury to the mucosa, and narrowing of the anastomosis with sloughing of devitalized cartilage can all impair pulmonary hygiene and secretion clearance, leading to the high incidence of bacterial infections after lung transplantation.

Secondary to inadequate secretion clearance, bronchoscopy is a valuable therapeutic tool in the postoperative period; this is discussed below (therapeutic bronchoscopy). Of note, the blunted cough reflex among lung transplant patients can have an advantage, reducing the amount of topical anesthesia needed within the airway. However, it is important to note that, among patients with a single lung transplant, the cough reflex is intact in the native lung.

Bacterial infections are the most common infectious complication, with 43%–63% of infections following lung transplant secondary to bacterial pathogens; however, viral (23%–31%), fungal (10%–14%), and other (4%–10%) opportunistic pathogens – including mycobacterial disease, *Nocardia*, *Actinomyces*, *Legionella*, and *Listeria monocytogenes* – must be considered.

Although routine Gram stain and culture are essential components to the evaluation of a change in clinical status, specimens must be targeted to a broad differential based on the presentation and other risk factors and/or exposures for a given patient. *Aspergillus* is commonly isolated during bronchoscopy among lung transplant patients but may be transient and associated with necrotic tissue found at the anastomotic site without true invasion. (*Pneumocystis carinii* is a potential opportunist infection following lung transplantation but has been virtually eliminated by the routine use of prophylaxis.) In the era before prophylaxis, infection was reported in up to 88% of heart or lung transplant recipients.

Even if bronchoscopy is performed, a pathogen is not always identified in the setting of clinical infection, secondary to initiating antibiotic treatment prior to the procedure. In addition, the sensitivity of bronchoscopy for diagnosing rejection is dependent on technique. In a study of bronchoscopy among patients with new respiratory symptoms using TBBx, BAL, and protected specimen brush (PSB), only 17.5% of bacterial infections were established using BAL; the diagnostic yield increased when using PSB.

Performing bronchoscopy in lung transplant patients is similar to that in nontransplant patients. Effective sedation is important to allow a safe and effective procedure. It is important to note patients with cystic fibrosis, who make up a significant proportion of lung transplant patients, tend to require higher doses of sedative medication for the procedure. Similar to bronchoscopy performed in nontransplant patients, complications of TBBx in lung transplant recipients include pneumothorax (1%–3%), pulmonary hemorrhage 10%–15%), arrhythmia (2%), upper airway obstruction requiring intervention (10%), and cardiopulmonary arrest and death (0.01%). As with any procedure, the risk of not performing a diagnostic procedure and proceeding without additional information that may influence management must be weighed against the risk of the procedure.

The risk of bleeding has been reported to be higher in lung transplant recipients compared with that reported in other populations and appears to be independent of traditional bleeding risks, including coagulation parameters, platelet count, serum creatinine, or use of aspirin or immunosuppressive drugs. It is also not correlated with the presence of acute rejection, BOS, the number of biopsies taken, or time since transplant. Improved bleeding rates among lung transplant patients has been shown after implementing a standardized protocol of (1) desmopressin for blood urea nitrogen >30, (2) avoidance of TBBx in patients with known pulmonary hypertension, and (3) withholding antiplatelet agents before the procedure. Some programs, including ours, perform all procedures using endotracheal intubation (without balloon deployed). This protocol can provide improved access to the airway during the procedure. In addition, it allows easy access to the airway for debridement when necessary in the early post-transplant period. Finally, lung transplant patients may be at higher risk for desaturation during the procedure, and performing the procedure following intubation can avoid upper airway obstruction, which is commonly implicated in desaturation events.

VISUALIZATION OF THE ANASTOMOSIS AND MANAGEMENT OF AIRWAY COMPLICATIONS

Bronchoscopy is the gold standard in the diagnosis of airway complications and is instrumental in their management. The most common anastomotic airway complications include stenosis, bronchomalacia, granulation tissue, anastomotic dehiscence, and anastomotic infections.

Airway complications are relatively common among lung transplant recipients, and diagnosis of a problem with the integrity of the anastomosis is critical in the management of a lung transplant recipient. Early studies suggested airway complication rates as high as 57%.

Changes in donor lung procurement, operative techniques, and postoperative management have improved this risk, resulting in lower rates of airway complications (12%–17%). The majority of airway complications involve the large central airways, in particular the bronchial anastomosis. The bronchial artery circulation is lost during the harvest of the donor lung, and limited bronchial artery revascularization from the recipient bronchial artery may take 3–4 weeks to occur after transplantation. During this time, the airway is dependent on retrograde low-pressure flow from the poorly oxygenated blood available in the pulmonary artery, and the risk of ischemia of the proximal donor bronchus (area just distal to the anastomosis in the recipient) is high. The majority of airways will display inflammation and erythema after transplantation and necrosis of some degree. The severity of this process correlates with the risk of serious airway complications. In the immediate postoperative period, bronchoscopy plays a role in monitoring the anastomosis and in helping with pulmonary hygiene and management of secretions. Early diagnosis of poor anastomotic healing can help in targeting a patient for close surveillance and determining the need for continued antimicrobial therapy secondary to airway infection. Changes in the innate defenses of lung transplant patients discussed above promote injury to the airway that can lead to an increased risk of infection. In addition, poor lymphatic drainage in the transplanted lung dictates that patients may require aggressive diuresis in the perioperative period; this can cause secretions to be thick and tenacious, making mobilization difficult. Bronchoscopy, during this early period, can help in the clearing of blood clots and thick tenacious secretions and in the debridement of necrotic tissue to help maintain a patent airway. In the majority of cases this can be performed with a flexible bronchoscope using a forceps. Less commonly, debridement in the operating room using laser, cryotherapy, or a rigid bronchoscope may be necessary.

Airway Stenosis

Stenosis is a late complication secondary to healing of early anastomotic injury or as a result of chronic rejection. Furthermore, airway narrowing may cause secretion retention, which may predispose to recurrent infections and progressive airway injury. The management of bronchial stenosis includes mechanical dilation, stenting, and bronchoscopic airway debridement using laser or cryotherapy. Mechanical dilation commonly requires serial procedures, and most centers would recommend dilation on at least two occasions prior to considering stent placement. Dilation allows for better evaluation of the extent of the stenosis and the airways distal to the narrowing. In addition, if the stenosis is secondary to either infection or inflammation of the airway, serial dilations may allow improved airway function while the primary process (infection or rejection) is aggressively treated. This may improve the long-term result and, in many cases, avoid stent placement. There is debate regarding the ideal stent for placement in stenotic airways. Silicone stents commonly require rigid bronchoscopy for placement. However, they have the advantage of easy removal to allow for further dilation. In addition, during serial dilations increasingly larger stents may be placed. The disadvantage of silicone stents is that they are prone to problems with secretion clearance and plugging. In contrast, self-expandable metallic stents can be used using a flexible bronchoscope but can exacerbate the fibrosis and granulation response of the airway, and metallic stents are extremely difficult to remove after being placed.

Segmental nonanastomotic bronchial stenosis or bronchomalacia can be seen in persons with infectious complications or in patients with multiple bouts of acute airway rejection. Treatment of the underlying infection or rejection is key to managing these complications and may result in resolution of the stenosis. Alternatively, mechanical dilation can be performed; less commonly, there can be stent placement if the airway is proximal and large enough to allow successful placement.

Bronchomalacia

Bronchomalacia can occur in combination with bronchial stenosis or independently and is also commonly associated with recurrent bronchial infection and/or rejection. Although bronchomalacia does not respond to balloon dilation, stent placement may improve airway patency.

Granulation Tissue

Granulation tissue can form in response to prior injury or secondary to a foreign body reaction. The suture material present at the anastomosis can stimulate a granulation tissue response. If airway obstruction is present secondary to granulation tissue, debridement using cryotherapy or local injection of corticosteroids is used. The use of a laser may cause thermal burns deep beneath the mucosal tissues and induce more scarring and granulation tissue formation or stenosis and should be used with caution.

Anastomotic Dehiscence

Incomplete or partial dehiscence can be managed conservatively with frequent bronchoscopies (to clear blood and necrotic tissue) along with antibiotic therapy. In some cases, temporary stenting may stabilize the airway to allow healing. However, stenting should not be performed in the presence of an active infection. As surgical technique has improved, the incidence of dehiscence has been decreasing; this is a rare complication in current practice.

Anastomotic Infections

Bacterial or fungal infections of the bronchial anastomosis are associated with poor healing. These infections are commonly polymicrobial. Treatment includes bronchoscopic debridement, which often requires serial procedures over long periods of time, in combination with aggressive antimicrobial therapy to achieve adequate control. Long-term sequelae including stenosis or bronchomalacia may occur that require dilation or stenting. However, placement of a stent is not recommended acutely until the infection is under control or (ideally) totally resolved.

Acknowledgements: Dr. Hilary Goldberg for review and editing of the content of this chapter.

LEARNING POINTS

1. Bronchoscopy is a pivotal procedure in the management of lung transplant patients.
2. There are four main indications for bronchoscopy following lung transplantation:
   a. Immediately after anastomosis to evaluate integrity of the airway
   b. Surveillance bronchoscopy with TBBx for rejection
   c. Diagnostic bronchoscopy for changes in clinical status
   d. Visualization of the anastomosis and management of airway complications including airway debridement, dilation, and/or stent placement
3. The performance of bronchoscopy in the lung transplant patient is the same as that in nontransplant patients, although some differences should be noted:
   a. The immunocompromised status of the patients widens the differential of potential pathogens that may cause infectious complications
   b. In lung transplant patients the cough reflex is blunted, which influences the risk of silent aspiration but can also improve tolerance of the procedure
   c. Some reports suggest an increased risk of bleeding with TBBx independent of other known bleeding risks, but the procedure can be safely and effectively performed in the patient population
4. There is debate among transplant centers regarding the utility of performing routine surveillance bronchoscopy with TBBx among lung transplant patients.

SUGGESTED READINGS

Alexander BD, Tapson VF. Infectious complications of lung transplantation. *Transplant Infect Dis.* 2001; 3(3):128–137.

Angel LF, Susanto I. Airway complications in lung transplantation. In: Lynch JP, Ross DJ, eds. *Lung and Heart Lung Transplantation.* Lung Biology in Health and Disease Series, Vol. 217, 1st ed. London: Taylor & Francis; 2006.

Cooper JD, Patterson GA, Trulock EP. Results of single and bilateral lung transplantation in 131 consecutive recipients. Washington University Lung Transplant Group. *J Thorac Cardiovasc Surg.* 1994;107(2):460–470; discussion 470–471.

De Vito Dabbs A, Hoffman LA, Iacono AT, et al. Are symptom reports useful for differentiating between acute rejection and pulmonary infection after lung transplantation? *Heart Lung.* 2004;33(6):372–380.

Diette GB, Wiener CM, White P. The higher risk of bleeding in lung transplant recipients from bronchoscopy is independent of traditional bleeding risks: results of a prospective cohort study. *Chest.* 1999;115(2):397–402.

Dransfield MT, Garver RI, Weill D. Standardized guidelines for surveillance bronchoscopy to reduce complication in lung transplant recipients. *J Heart Lung Transplant.* 2004;23(1):110–114.

Griffith BP, Zenati M. The pulmonary donor. *Clin Chest Med.* 1990;11(2):217–226.

Guilinger RA, Paradis IL, Dauber JH, et al. The importance of bronchoscopy with transbronchial biopsy and bronchoalveolar lavage in the management of lung transplant recipients. *Am J Respir Crit Care Med.* 1995;152(6 Pt 1):2037–2043.

Kramer MR, Marshall SE, Starnes VA, Gamberg P, Amitai Z, Theodore J. Infectious complications in heart-lung transplantation. Analysis of 200 episodes. *Arch Intern Med.* 1993;153(17):2010–2016.

Kukafka DS, O'Brien GM, Furukawa S, Criner GJ. Surveillance bronchoscopy in lung transplant recipients. *Chest.* 1997;111(2):377–381.

Levine SM. Transplant/Immunology Network of the American College of Chest Physicians. A survey of clinical practice of lung transplantation in North America. *Chest.* 2004;125(4):1224–1238.

Orens JB, Estenne M, Arcasoy S, et al. Pulmonary Scientific Council of the International Society for Heart and Lung Transplantation. International guidelines for the selection of lung transplant candidates: 2006 update–a consensus report from the Pulmonary Scientific Council of the International Society for Heart and Lung Transplantation. *J Heart Lung Transplant.* 2006;25(7):745–755.

Pomerance A, Madden B, Buke MM, Yacoub MH. Transbronchial biopsy in heart and lung transplantation: clinicopathologic correlations. *J Heart Lung Transplant.* 1995;14(4):761–773.

Riou B, Guesde R, Jacquens Y, Duranteau R, Viars P. Fiberoptic bronchoscopy in brain-dead organ donors. *Am J Respir Crit Care Med.* 1994;150(2):558–560.

Shennib H, Massard G. Airway complications in lung transplantation. *Ann Thorac Surg.* 1994;57:506–551.

Tiroke AH, Bewig B, Haverich A. Bronchoalveolar lavage in lung transplantation. State of the art. *Clin Transplant.* 1999;13(2):131–157.

Trulock EP, Ettinger NA, Brunt EM, Pasque MK, Kaiser LR, Cooper JD. The role of transbronchial lung biopsy in the treatment of lung transplant recipients. An analysis of 200 consecutive procedures. *Chest.* 1992;102(4):1049–1054.

Valentine VG, Taylor DE, Dhillon GS, et al. Success of lung transplantation without surveillance bronchoscopy. *J Heart Lung Transplant.* 2002;21(3):319–326.

Wahidi MM, Ernst A. The role of bronchoscopy in the management of lung transplant recipients. *Respir Care Clin.* 2004;10:549–562.

Yousem SA. Significance of clinically silent untreated mild acute cellular rejection in lung allograft recipients. *Hum Pathol.* 1996;27(3):269–273.

Yousem SA, Berry GJ, Cagle PT, et al. Revision of the 1990 working formulation for the classification of pulmonary allograft rejection: Lung Rejection Study Group. *J Heart Lung Transplant.* 1996;15(1 Pt 1):1–15.

Yousem SA, Paradis I, Griffith BP. Can transbronchial biopsy aid in the diagnosis of bronchiolitis obliterans in lung transplant recipients? *Transplantation.* 1994;57(1):151–153.

14

ADVANCED DIAGNOSTIC BRONCHOSCOPY

Ross Morgan and Armin Ernst

Over the past decade a range of new diagnostic tools has become available to the bronchoscopist, and this range reflects technological advancements such as the development of miniaturized transducers as well as advanced image guidance. Many of these techniques have yet to find an established role in practice and remain research tools. Others, in particular endobronchial ultrasound (EBUS) guidance, have had an immediate clinical impact and are now considered state-of-the-art technologies. The tools discussed below can be broadly grouped together into two categories based on their utility. The first group is used to extend the diagnostic reach of the bronchoscope to direct biopsy of distal lesions or lesions outside the airway and includes EBUS, ultrathin, and electromagnetic navigational bronchoscopy (ENB). The second broad category includes tools such as autofluorescence bronchoscopy (AFB), narrow band imaging (NBI), and high-magnification videobronchoscopy, which primarily aim to improve detection rates for the preinvasive bronchial lesions of dysplasia and carcinoma in situ (CIS). Such lesions, which are only a few cell layers thick, are often missed on regular white light bronchoscopy.

ENDOBRONCHIAL ULTRASOUND

EBUS technology has probably been the greatest advance in diagnostic bronchoscopy since the widespread introduction of the flexible bronchoscope (FB) in the 1960s. It provides the enormous advantage of allowing the endoscopist to look within, as well as outside, the airway wall, is safe and noninvasive for patients, and is relatively straightforward to use. There are currently two types of probe in use: the radial scanning ultrasound probe and the dedicated linear-array EBUS bronchoscope.

The radial scanning ultrasound probe is a miniaturized probe that is passed through the working channel of the FB. The probe consists of a rotating piezoelectric crystal that acts as both a signal generator and receiver of ultrasound waves (Figure 14.1). As the crystal rotates, a 360° picture is displayed. A water-filled balloon, inflated after passage of the probe through the working channel of the bronchoscope, allows coupling of the ultrasound waves to the airway wall. The frequency of this EBUS probe is 20 MHz; this allows very high-resolution (<1-mm) images and excellent assessment of the layers of the airway wall and peribronchial structures adjacent to the bronchi within the mediastinum (Figure 14.2). Its ability to define the bronchial wall layers makes it an excellent tool in distinguishing extrinsic compression from tissue invasion in the assessment of lung tumors. It has been found to be more sensitive than computed tomography (CT) for this purpose, and its findings correlate very closely to surgical pathology findings. Other applications for investigating the structure of the

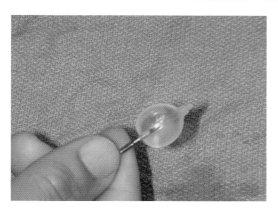

FIGURE 14.1. Tip of the radial ultrasound probe and sheath. The water-filled balloon allows for coupling of the device to the airway wall and facilitates ultrasound transmission.

airway wall include staging of CIS of the tracheobronchial tree and planning interventional procedures in the patient with airway obstruction. Especially in assessing patients with airway CIS who are planning to undergo photodynamic therapy, careful EBUS staging is now considered a requirement by most authorities in the field to decrease the likelihood for recurrences after endobronchial treatment.

An expanding role for the radial EBUS probe is in increasing the yield of flexible bronchoscopy in the diagnosis of peripheral lung lesions and solitary pulmonary nodules. For this purpose, the EBUS probe is inserted through a guide sheath

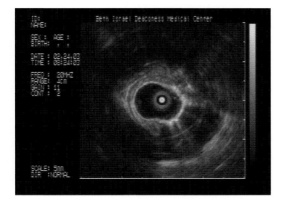

FIGURE 14.2. Radial EBUS image of the left main stem bronchus. The airway wall at the superior aspect is thickened from a small non-small cell lung cancer.

into the bronchus leading to the segment where the lesion is suspected to be found based on the preprocedure CT scan. The area of interest is seen as a dark homogenous lesion within the "snowstorm-like" ultrasound appearance of normal alveolar tissue. When this target is reached, the probe is removed and a biopsy forceps passed out through the guide sheath. The diagnostic yield for EBUS-guided biopsy of peripheral lung lesions is reported to be from 58.3% to 80% and recently has been shown to be increased further by use of a multimodality approach in combination with ENB to as high as 88%, a yield that was independent of lesion size or lobar location. A further use of the radial EBUS probe is in the evaluation of central mediastinal lesions. As it gives good resolution up to a depth of 5 cm, this EBUS probe has been found to be helpful in localizing and guiding transbronchial needle aspirations (TBNAs) from enlarged structures adjacent to the bronchi within the mediastinum nodes where it increases the diagnostic yield of TBNA from malignant lymph nodes, in particular from sites other than the central mediastinum, below the carina. In the last couple of years, however, the role of the radial probe for this purpose has been largely superseded by the dedicated linear array EBUS bronchoscope (EBUS-TBNA scope).

The EBUS-TBNA scope is a completely different system from the radial system discussed earlier. It is architecturally similar to the dedicated endoscopic ultrasound-fine needle aspiration (EUS-FNA) endoscopes used in gastroenterology. These EUS-FNA endoscopes permit biopsy of mediastinal lesions using the esophagus as the conduit. The EBUS-TBNA scope is smaller than its gastroenterological cousin, but looks similar. A convex array digital ultrasound transducer is mounted at the distal tip (Figure 14.3). The bronchoscope has an outer diameter of 6.9 mm, a 2.0-mm instrument channel, and viewing optics that are at a 30° oblique angle. Scanning is performed at a frequency of 7.5 MHz and to a depth of 50 mm. This frequency does not allow for the same resolution as the radial probe; therefore, the scope is not used for

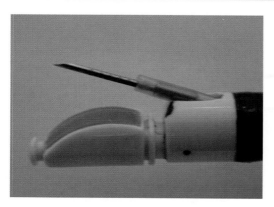

FIGURE 14.3. Distal tip of a dedicated EBUS scope to facilitate transbronchial needle aspiration under real-time vision. The view and working channel have an oblique orientation.

diagnostic ultrasound evaluations, but merely for procedural guidance. Similarly, the endoscopic image is suboptimal compared with those of conventional bronchoscopes, and, for a full airway evaluation, conventional bronchoscopy needs to be performed separately. Using the EBUS-TBNA scope can be a challenge for the bronchoscopist who is used to the forward view only, in particular for passing though the vocal cords.

This instrument is an excellent tool for lymph node puncture, with diagnostic yields that are equivalent to and may even surpass those obtained at surgical mediastinoscopy mainly because of its ability to reach nodal groups not accessible by the surgical route. Two images are provided, one of the airway, and the other an ultrasound image. When the node of interest is located on the ultrasound image, a color Doppler function allows confirmation of vessels before node sampling is performed. A dedicated 22-gauge needle with a stylet is passed through the working channel and exits the distal end of the bronchoscope at a 20° angle. A protective sheath is first advanced and is visualized on the airway view and locked in place. Following this, the needle is pushed into the lymph node under real-time ultrasound guidance, the stylet is removed, and aspirates are taken. Studies suggest that, in combination with EUS, complete mediastinal staging (vital in therapeutic planning

for lung cancer) can be achieved noninvasively with EBUS. These exciting results suggest that this bronchoscope has the potential to truly revolutionize the staging algorithm for non-small cell lung cancer.

There is a long learning curve for training in the use of the radial EBUS probe. The biggest challenge for the bronchoscopist is becoming accustomed to a 360° ultrasonic view of the bronchial anatomy that, when the probe is distal to the midline trachea, is visualized at an oblique angle, rather than as the familiar axial view on the CT scan. As a result, it is suggested that approximately 50 ultrasound examinations are required to achieve proficiency with this probe. The learning curve for facility with the puncture scope is steeper, particularly for those already familiar with TBNA.

ULTRATHIN BRONCHOSCOPY

The bronchial tree in the human may divide up to 20 times before the respiratory bronchioles are reached. The view from the standard FB (with an external diameter of around 6 mm) is typically limited to the first three to four divisions of the tree. Ultrathin bronchoscopes (with external diameters of 2.8 mm) can be guided under direct vision to a median of the sixth generation bronchi (range, fourth- to ninth-generation bronchi), allowing more distal examination, and have been used in conjunction with virtual bronchoscopy navigation for small peripheral pulmonary lesions. A major limitation of this system is the lack of a good size working channel through which to obtain biopsies and the difficulty to maintain proper orientation within the distal bronchial tree. Studies trying to establish the exact place for this technology are ongoing.

ELECTROMAGNETIC NAVIGATIONAL BRONCHOSCOPY

As outlined in other chapters, one of the biggest challenges in bronchoscopy is the reliable biopsy

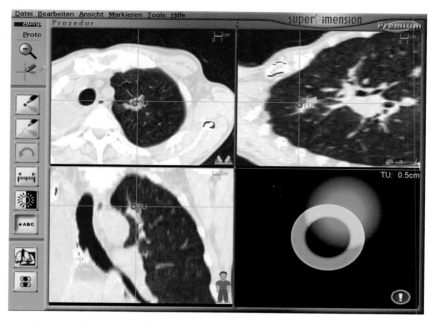

FIGURE 14.4. Screen shot of ENB. One can see the relationship of the navigational tool to the identified lesion in several planes. *Bottom right*: Information about distance and directionality.

of peripheral lesions, which historically has been problematic with yields reported to be as low as 10%. Traditionally, transbronchial biopsy has been performed without any imaging guidance in diffuse processes, or fluoroscopy for specific lesions. A newer development is ENB, which has been used successfully in the last few years to improve the diagnostic approach to peripheral lesions.

Advanced CT imaging (as described in another chapter) has been innovatively combined with an electromagnetic navigation system to guide the bronchoscopic biopsy of peripheral lung nodules that lie beyond the reach of a standard bronchoscope. This technology involves placing the patient on a low-field, electromagnetic location board, thereby creating an electromagnetic field around the chest. A number of registration points are chosen on the CT image and then on the body as coordinates, and the system marries the two to provide a CT roadmap. A position sensor is incorporated into the distal end of a flexible catheter, which also serves

as an extended working channel for access of bronchoscopic tools. When this dedicated localization tool is placed within the electromagnetic field, the orientation and position of the sensor within the x, y, and z planes can be registered by use of specially designed computer software. This localizing sensor information is displayed on a monitor in real time and is subsequently mapped and superimposed on previously acquired multidetector CT images, thereby allowing for simultaneous virtual and active image guidance. The instruments that are sensor equipped are in fact steerable, which in itself is a difference from conventional tools used in bronchoscopy. When the sensor reaches the target lesion, the sensor probe is removed, and flexible forceps, brushes, or needles can be advanced precisely into the lesion for sampling (Figure 14.4).

Results suggest that the realistic success rate of biopsies of peripheral lesions is 55%–75% with this technique. The incidence of pneumothorax is in the region of 5%–8%, which is considerably lower than that following percutaneous biopsy. An additional advantage over CT guidance is that there is no radiation exposure to patient and staff during the procedure. The principal hurdles in the use of ENB at present are the added time it takes to perform the procedure (about 10 minutes in well-trained hands) and dislodgment of the catheters when biopsy instruments are introduced, resulting in a nondiagnostic procedure. Additional restraints are the inability to directly visualize the lesion prior to biopsy and the cost of the system. In many institutions, ENB is often combined with radial EBUS imaging for the biopsy of peripheral lesions. This study found the highest diagnostic yields when both were used (88%) compared with yields when either technique was used alone.

Overall, this technology is still new and not yet firmly established. Every bronchoscopist also needs to remember that not every peripheral lesion requires biopsy. Some can be followed longitudinally, and in other circumstances it may be more adequate and cost effective to proceed with primary resection or another procedure, such as mediastinal biopsies in patients with peripheral lesions and mediastinal lymphadenopathy.

AUTOFLUORESCENCE BRONCHOSCOPY

Conventional white light bronchoscopy uses the full visible wavelength range (400–700 nm) to illuminate the mucosal surface; light is reflected, backscattered, or absorbed to produce an image. Normal respiratory tissue fluoresces green when exposed to light in the violet–blue spectrum (400–450 nm) because of the activation of cellular chromophores. Diseased tissue is associated with a change in the biochemical structure of the chromophores within the cells as well as with alterations in cell morphology and epithelial thickness that affect this green fluorescence. The utility of AFB is based on the observation that, as disease of the mucosa progresses along the spectrum from dysplasia to CIS, there

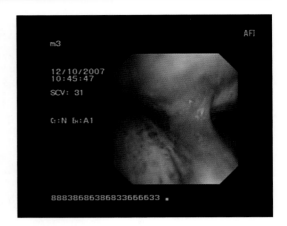

FIGURE 14.5. Image of a main carina as seen on AFB. The *greenish* color represents normal epithelium. The *pinkish* color is consistent with an early-stage carcinoma.

is a progressive loss of green autofluorescence, causing a red–brown appearance of the tissue (Figure 14.5). AFB has been shown to increase the diagnostic accuracy for squamous dysplasia and CIS when used in conjunction with conventional bronchoscopy, with studies suggesting that white light bronchoscopy alone detects, on average, only 40% of high-grade dysplasia and CIS, with an increased detection rate to 88% with AFB. It should be noted, however, that many of the studies compared AFB to fiber-optic bronchoscopy, the image quality from which is inferior to that obtained with newer videobronchoscopes, now widely in use. Although the technique is easy to learn, it does require some time to become familiar with it. The examination is performed before other interventions, and excessive suctioning needs to be avoided as the resultant airway wall trauma makes the examination difficult to interpret. The major downside to AFB apart from cost is the low specificity as differentiating preinvasive lesions from bronchitis is problematic, resulting in many false-positive findings. In addition, the utility of this procedure is undermined by the fact that now there is no widely accepted algorithm on the management of the lesions that it detects.

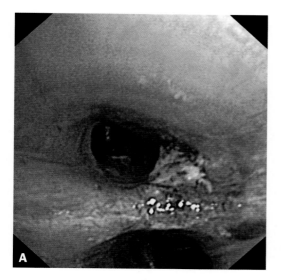
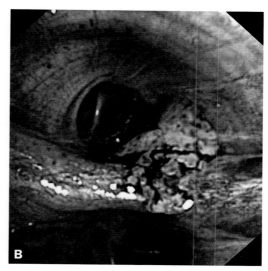

FIGURE 14.6. Conventional imaging of a carinal squamous cell cancer **(A)**. Same image obtained through NBI **(B)**. Observe the superior imaging of the vasculature.

HIGH-MAGNIFICATION VIDEOBRONCHOSCOPY AND NARROW BAND IMAGING

Changes in blood vessel number, size, and complexity are associated with premalignant and cancerous lesions. NBI technology, in use for some time in GI endoscopy, is used to detect vessel growth and complex vessel networks in the bronchial mucosa, and may be useful to detect these lesions. Blood vessel enhancement is achieved by use of the light absorption characteristics of hemoglobin at specific wavelengths. Two narrow band filters are used, one to detect 415-nm light that is absorbed by surface level capillaries, and a second to detect 540-nm light that is absorbed by vessels below the surface layer (Figure 14.6, A and B). This permits visualization of abnormal distribution and dilatation of blood vessels in the mucosa and, in combination with high-magnification videobronchoscopy (up to 110×), yields clear images of the microvasculature. NBI is likely to be of value in combination with other modalities but awaits a classification method in the airway. AFB and NBI can be thought of as complementary tools; AFB serves as the screening tool, followed by a focused mucosal examination with NBI. It is expected that a videobronchoscope that combines both modalities will be shortly available.

OTHER TECHNOLOGIES THAT AWAIT VALIDATION BUT THAT HAVE BEEN USED IN HUMAN RESEARCH: OPTICAL COHERENCE TOMOGRAPHY AND CONFOCAL MICROENDOSCOPY

The latter uses a 1-mm probe, which is passed through the FB working channel and placed in direct contact with the airway wall, providing high-definition microscopic imaging of the mucosal surface at resolutions of 5 mm. While this technology awaits validation and assessment of clinical utility, it offers the exciting potential of extending the reach of the FB to the distal end of the bronchial tree to provide dynamic imaging of the terminal bronchioles and alveoli.

Simulation Technology

One major obstacle in the introduction of new technologies and their safe use is the fact that most training programs do not routinely offer them; therefore, exposure and practice are limited. Only a few interventional training programs are active in the United States, and their numbers are insufficient to train significant numbers of interested pulmonologists.

Simulation technology is gaining increasing attention in the medical community. Long incorporated into military and flight training, simulation technology has also been a cornerstone of anesthesia and surgical training (especially since the introduction of minimally invasive surgery) in many institutions. Simulation allows for the training of complex or high-risk procedures in a low-stress environment and can be repeated as often as necessary. This is in contrast to the conventional apprentice model of training in which the procedure volume cannot be controlled, steps cannot be repeated, and the procedure has to be practiced by a novice on patients.

Simulation is available for technical skill training as well as team training (e.g., code situations) and decision making. Simulation can be very high tech as is the case in the creation of computer-based virtual environments (high-fidelity simulation), or rather low tech (low-fidelity simulation), such as practicing thoracoscopy in a cardboard box. Virtual reality simulation is more "lifelike," but not necessarily superior in efficacy to low-fidelity simulation, depending on the specific task.

Simulation training holds great promise for the education of the professional interested in acquiring new skills, and research in the field of bronchoscopy is growing. We should also be prepared that it may be introduced into ongoing competency assessment and proficiency evaluations, as it is in the case of pilots. Regional simulation centers could assume roles of competency assessment and evelution of proficiency, and it is our opinion that simulation holds great promise for the future of skills training and assessment in bronchoscopy.

SUGGESTED READINGS

Eberhardt R, Anantham D, Ernst A, Feller-Kopman D, Herth F. Multimodality bronchoscopic diagnosis of peripheral lung lesions: a randomized controlled trial. *Am J Respir Crit Care Med.* 2007;176(1):36–41. Epub 2007 Mar 22.

Eberhardt R, Anantham D, Herth F, et al. Electromagnetic navigation diagnostic bronchoscopy in peripheral lung lesions. *Chest.* 2007;131(6):1800–1805. Epub 2007 Mar 30.

Ernst A, Silvestri GA, Johnstone D. Interventional pulmonary procedures: guidelines from the American College of Chest Physicians. *Chest.* 2003;123(5):1693–1717.

Feller-Kopman D, Lunn W, Ernst A. Autofluorescence bronchoscopy and endobronchial ultrasound: a practical review. *Ann Thorac Surg.* 2005;80(6):2395–2401.

Gildea TR, Mazzone PJ, Karnak D, et al. Electromagnetic navigation diagnostic bronchoscopy: a prospective study. *Am J Respir Crit Care Med.* 2006;174(9):982–989.

Herth F, Becker HD, Ernst A. Conventional vs endobronchial ultrasound-guided transbronchial needle aspiration: a randomized trial. *Chest.* 2004;125(1):322–325.

Herth F, Ernst A, Schulz M, et al. Endobronchial ultrasound reliably differentiates between airway infiltration and compression by tumor. *Chest.* 2003;123(2):458–462.

Herth FJ, Eberhardt R, Vilmann P, et al. Real-time endobronchial ultrasound guided transbronchial needle aspiration for sampling mediastinal lymph nodes. *Thorax.* 2006;61(9):795–798.

Herth FJ, Ernst A, Becker HD. Endobronchial ultrasound-guided transbronchial lung biopsy in solitary pulmonary nodules and peripheral lesions. *Eur Respir J.* 2002;20(4):972–974.

Herth FJ, Rabe KF, Gasparini S, et al. Transbronchial and transoesophageal (ultrasound-guided) needle aspirations for the analysis of mediastinal lesions. *Eur Respir J.* 2006;28(6):1264–1275.

Kurimoto N, Miyazawa T, Okimasa S, et al. Endobronchial ultrasonography using a guide sheath increases the ability to diagnose peripheral pulmonary lesions endoscopically. *Chest.* 2004;126(3):959–965.

Lam S, MacAulay C, leRiche JC, et al. Detection and localization of early lung cancer by fluorescence bronchoscopy. *Cancer.* 2000;89(11 Suppl):2468–2473.

Paone G, Nicastri E, Lucantoni G, et al. Endobronchial ultrasound-driven biopsy in the diagnosis
of peripheral lung lesions. *Chest.* 2005;128(5):3551–
3557.

Richards-Kortum R, Sevick-Muraca E. Quantitative optical spectroscopy for tissue diagnosis. *Annu Rev Phys
Chem.* 1996;47:555–606.

Thiberville L, Moreno-Swirc S, Vercauteren T, et al. In
vivo imaging of the bronchial wall microstructure
using fibered confocal fluorescence microscopy. *Am
J Respir Crit Care Med.* 2007;175(1):22–31.

Vincent BD, Fraig M, Silvestri GA. A pilot study of narrow
band imaging compared to white light bronchoscopy
for evaluation of normal airways, pre-malignant and
malignant airways disease. *Chest.* 2007;131(6):1794–
1799. Epub 2007 May 15.

Yasufuku K, Nakajima T, Motoori K, et al. Comparison of
endobronchial ultrasound, positron emission tomography, and CT for lymph node staging of lung cancer.
Chest. 2006;130(3):710–718.

15

BASIC THERAPEUTIC TECHNIQUES

Luis F. Angel and Deborah J. Levine

INTRODUCTION

Interventional pulmonology is an evolving discipline stemming from pulmonary medicine that concentrates on both diagnostic and therapeutic interventions for patients with advanced airway and pleural diseases. The interventional pulmonologist has taken an active role in developing potentially less invasive ways to perform diagnostic and therapeutic procedures in disorders of the airway and pleura.

Procedures encompassed within this expanding field include, but are not limited to, rigid bronchoscopy, endobronchial laser therapy, electrocautery, cryotherapy, balloon dilation (BD), brachytherapy (BT), and endotracheal or endobronchial stent placement. The question of which modality to use is influenced by many factors, including patient presentation, operator proficiency, anesthetic techniques, and the institution's available equipment. The key to success in caring for patients with these disorders is careful patient selection and the complementary application of these techniques. In this review we will focus on describing these procedures, as well as outlining an active approach to the clinical disorders for which they are used.

CENTRAL AIRWAYS OBSTRUCTION

Obstruction or stenosis of the trachea and large bronchi can be a consequence of endobronchial obstruction, extraluminal compression, or a combination of both. Endoluminal or endobronchial lesions are most common. Extrinsic compression causing obstruction of the airway is less frequent, but can result in symptoms and outcomes similar to those of endobronchial obstruction. Most cases are secondary to bronchogenic carcinoma; however, both benign and malignant causes can produce significant morbidity and decreased life expectancy if left untreated. Table 15.1 shows the common etiologies of central airway obstruction.

The presenting symptoms of airway obstruction will differ depending on the anatomic location and severity of the obstruction. Symptoms range from chronic hoarseness, cough, dyspnea, and wheezing to more severe acute problems such as stridor, hemoptysis, and respiratory failure. When approaching the patient with upper airway obstruction, the pulmonologist must take into account the stability of the patient, the underlying pathologic condition, and the short- and long-term prognoses of the disease process. The location and severity of the lesion and the

Table 15.1. *Conditions associated with central airway obstruction*

Malignant	Nonmalignant
Primary endoluminal carcinoma:	Lymphadenopathy:
Bronchogenic	Sarcoidosis
Adenoid cystic	Infectious (i.e., tuberculosis)
Mucoepidermoid	Vascular:
Carcinoid	Sling
Metastatic carcinoma to the airway:	Cartilage:
Bronchogenic	Relapsing polychondritis
Renal cell	Granulation tissue from:
Breast	Endotracheal tubes
Thyroid	Tracheostomy tubes
Colon	Airway stents
Sarcoma	Foreign bodies
Melanoma	Surgical anastomoses
Laryngeal carcinoma	Wegener's granulomatosis
Esophageal carcinoma	Pseudotumor:
Mediastinal tumors:	Hamartomas
Thymus	Amyloid
Thyroid	Papillomatosis
Germ cell	Hyperdynamic:
Lymphadenopathy associated with any of the	Tracheomalacia
above malignancies:	Bronchomalacia
Lymphoma	Other:
	Goiter
	Mucus plug
	Vocal cord paralysis
	Epiglottitis
	Blood clot

rate of progression of the obstruction are significant aspects that need to be considered when evaluating these difficult conditions. The availability of equipment and the expertise of the interventionalist are also important factors in deciding how to treat the individual patient. Most patients will require a combination of various techniques for the most successful outcomes.

RIGID BRONCHOSCOPY

The rigid bronchoscope is an invaluable tool that allows the interventional pulmonologist to secure, evaluate, and manipulate the trachea and proximal bronchi, while controlling oxygenation and ventilation. It is the most rapid technique to relieve an obstruction of the central airways, whether it is an intraluminal or extraluminal obstruction.

Today, a majority of bronchoscopies are being performed with the flexible scope; making it the procedure of choice for most diagnostic and some therapeutic procedures. Despite this rapid expansion and widespread use of the flexible scope, however, the rigid scope still remains an imperative tool for therapeutic practice. Both flexible and rigid bronchoscopy have unique characteristics and offer specific advantages depending on the clinical situation. Table 15.2 compares rigid and flexible bronchoscopy and the best indications for specific clinical scenarios.

Table 15.2. *Comparison of rigid and flexible bronchoscopy*

	Rigid bronchoscopy	Flexible bronchoscopy
Expertise	7% of practicing pulmonologists	95% of practicing pulmonologists
Anesthesia	General anesthesia	Conscious sedation
Oxygenation and ventilation	Excellent support for both with jet or conventional ventilation	Poor support for oxygenation and ventilation
Bleeding control	Better visualization and suctioning	Poor visualization and ineffective suction
Location of the lesion	Ideal for central and large airways lesions	Easy access to central and distal airways
Size of biopsies	Large	Small
Mechanical debridement	More effective and efficient	Less effective and time consuming
Foreign body removal	Easier and effective in large or central airways	Effective but may be more difficult and time consuming
Management of critical airway narrowing	Gold standard	May worsen airway obstruction
Dilatation of strictures	Mechanical dilation possible with the rigid scope	Possible with the use of balloon dilation

For patients with respiratory insufficiency secondary to central airways obstruction, re-establishment of the airway can be accomplished with intubation and advancement of the rigid scope. The airway can then be dilated by the advancement of the scope along the wall of the airway. This dilation may be temporary, but will allow oxygenation, ventilation, and time to evaluate the obstructed area for further therapy. If the airway is too narrow to allow advancement of the scope, balloons of increasing diameter can be passed through the scope for dilation. The scope can then be used as a tumor-debulking instrument, by "corkscrewing" the scope to core out large pieces of tumor. In patients with extrinsic compression causing airway obstruction, the rigid bronchoscope is required for the insertion of silicone stents in the trachea or proximal bronchi. Rigid bronchoscopy is also a vital tool in controlling massive hemoptysis. Hemorrhage can be controlled by tamponade with the scope and with the use of large suction catheters to remove blood or clots.

With proper technique and safe anesthesia, there are few complications associated with rigid bronchoscopy. The most common problems come during intubation or advancement of the scope, causing trauma to the teeth, oropharynx, trachea, or bronchial walls. Massive bleeding is rare. There are few contraindications to rigid bronchoscopy, and most are related to use of general anesthesia. These include unstable cardiopulmonary status and serious arrhythmias.

LASER

Laser therapy is the most commonly recognized endobronchial treatment that the interventional pulmonologist uses today. It is used extensively for the palliation of symptoms of airway obstruction secondary to malignancies, and it provides effective therapy for benign airway lesions and stenosis. In selected patients, laser therapy has been shown to improve quality of life and functional status, and, in some cases, to extend survival.

The most widely used laser in the tracheobronchial tree is the neodymium-doped yttrium aluminium garnet (Nd:YAG) laser because of its deep penetration into tissues (≤ 5 mm), superior coagulation characteristics, cutting ability, and versatility. It can be used through a flexible or rigid bronchoscope. The decision between using a flexible or rigid bronchoscope depends on the operator's experience, the character of the lesion, and patient stability. Lesions that are favorable to laser therapy include tracheal and main stem lesions, polypoid lesions of short length (<4 cm), lesions with a visible distal airway lumen, and functional lung distal to the obstruction. Lesions that are not favorable for laser resection have more than 80% obstruction of the airway and are those that destroy airway wall integrity and obliterate anatomical boundaries.

Palliation of symptoms from malignant airway obstruction is the most common indication for endobronchial laser therapy. It is also used for obstruction secondary to benign tumors such as hamartomas, papillomas, amyloidomas, and endobronchial endometriosis.

Bronchoscopic laser therapy is a relatively safe procedure. Most complications can be avoided by applying preventative safety measures. Perforation of a vascular structure, mediastinum, or esophagus is one of the most feared complications of laser therapy. Knowing the anatomic proximity of the aortic arch, pulmonary artery, and the esophagus is crucial when performing laser therapy near these areas. Another concerning complication is a laser-related endobronchial fire. Fires are uncommon when the rigid bronchoscope is used. Materials that ignite during laser therapy include the flexible scope sheath, endotracheal tubes, and silicone stents.

Contraindications to endobronchial laser therapy include extrinsic compression of the airway without an endobronchial lesion, involvement or compression of the pulmonary artery by tumor, tracheoesophageal fistula, and prolonged atelectasis for more than 4 weeks.

ELECTROCAUTERY AND ARGON PLASMA COAGULATION

Although the Nd:YAG laser is recognized as the most widely used form of bronchoscopic

intervention, its use may be limited by its expense, its relative lack of accessibility, and the belief that rigid bronchoscopy is required for its use. These factors have increased the appeal of a parallel procedure, electrocautery, which may be more available, more user friendly, and less expensive. Furthermore, there are many studies that present evidence that electrocautery has efficacy similar to that of laser therapy.

Bronchoscopic electrocautery, also called electrocoagulation (EC), unlike laser therapy, is usually performed in the contact mode, with the probe gently touching the tissue. A snare is available for polypoid lesions, and a standard probe is available for the bulky lesions. The indications, patient selection, and principles of application are essentially the same as for the Nd:YAG laser. Both benign and malignant lesions have proven to be amenable to electrocautery.

Complications are relatively similar to those of laser therapy, with hemorrhage, airway perforation, and (rarely) endobronchial fire. The EC probe needs to be cleaned from debris intermittently during the procedure, which is one disadvantage when comparing it with laser therapy. In general, however, EC has significant potential as an effective and cost-effective procedure for patients with endobronchial obstruction.

Argon plasma coagulation (APC) is a newer form of EC. It is used for both malignant and benign airway obstruction and endobronchial hemoptysis. It is used in the noncontact mode, similar to laser therapy. APC has the unique advantage of being able to treat lesions lateral to the probe. APC is less efficient than laser therapy at debulking large masses because it cannot generate as high of temperatures and provide as deep of tissue penetration.

CRYOTHERAPY

Cryotherapy refers to the use of extreme cold for medical therapy. The goal of cryotherapy is to destroy pathologic tissue, while preserving normal mucosa. The basis of action relies on destruction of tissue by repeated cycles of freezing and thawing. Nitrous oxide (N_2O) is the most common cryogen used in endobronchial therapy.

There are many factors that influence tissue injury when cryotherapy is used. The absolute temperature, the rate of cooling and thawing, and the length of freezing time all affect the success of therapy. Freezing to –40°C at the rate of −100°C/min has been shown to cause >90% cell death. Tissue vascularity, the distance of tissue from the probe, the amount of water in the tissue, and the number of freeze–thaw cycles have also been found to be essential factors in the effectiveness of the therapy. The destruction of tissue by freezing occurs by both an immediate and delayed mechanism.

Tissues are either cryosensitive or cryoresistant, which is why certain tissues respond better than others to cryotherapy. Skin, mucous membranes, and granulation tissue (which arises histologically from mucous membranes) are cryosensitive, whereas fat cartilage and fibrous and connective tissue are cryoresistant. Tumor cells have been found to be more cryosensitive than are normal cells, making cryotherapy an attractive therapy for endobronchial malignancies.

The indications for cryotherapy are similar to those for laser and EC; however, each type of therapy has unique properties that may make one indicated over another in specific cases. Cryotherapy has been used most often for local therapy in the palliation of airway malignancies, and is also successfully used in benign airway conditions. It is effective in treating airway stenosis caused by excessive granulation tissue after lung transplant, and was reported to decrease the percentage of patients who required stent placement. Cryotherapy is excellent for papillomas as they are quite cryosensitive. It is successful in removing foreign bodies from the airway, especially objects that are friable or tend to fall apart with forceps. The object is frozen and then removed from the patient's airway with the probe and scope as one unit. This technique can also

be used when removing blood clots and mucous plugs. Cryotherapy can decrease the risk of hemorrhage if performed prior to the biopsy of a suspected carcinoid lesion.

The lesions best treated with cryotherapy (whether they are benign or malignant) tend to be polypoid in nature and short in length, and they have a large endobronchial component. Long tapering lesions, bulky endobronchial lesions, or those with extensive submucosal involvement are not as favorable. Cryotherapy offers no benefit to patients with obstruction from pure extrinsic compression of the airway.

The advantages of cryotherapy are that it is a procedure that is easy to learn, relatively inexpensive (as compared with laser therapy), and safe. In comparison with laser or electrocautery, it does not have the danger of causing endobronchial fire. It is superior to modalities for distal lesions, as the risk of airway perforation is much lower. The cryoresistance of the bronchial tissue surrounding the lesions explains the safety of using cryotherapy. The main disadvantage of cryotherapy is that its effects are not immediate. It can take up to 2–4 weeks to show its maximum benefit and usually requires repeated bronchoscopies for follow-up and retreatment.

BALLOON DILATION

In the past, non-emergent cases of airway stenosis have been treated by introducing rigid bronchoscopes of increasing diameters or by dilation by semirigid dilator. These techniques have been largely replaced by the use of BD performed using either rigid or flexible bronchoscopy. BD is an effective procedure to restore patency of airways that are narrowed from either benign or malignant processes. The great benefit of BD is that it is a relatively nontraumatic and rapid procedure to use in airway strictures. It is most frequently used in combination with other endobronchial techniques, but may be used alone in selected cases.

The balloon catheter is passed through the working channel of the bronchoscope or threaded over a guide wire (using the Seldinger method) and placed across the stenosis, with the balloon protruding slightly beyond either end. The balloon, which is slightly larger than the stenotic area, is then gradually inflated with water for 30–120 seconds at increasing pressures. Fluoroscopy has traditionally been used to monitor the inflation, but has been shown to be unnecessary when the stenotic region is visualized bronchoscopically. Serial dilations are performed with the same balloon or with one of a larger diameter until the airway lumen is restored. It is best to be able to visualize the airway distal to the stenosis to assess which size balloon should be used. This therapy has been shown to be best suited for stenotic areas that are short in length. Patients with transmural strictures that occupy a long segment of the airway usually require either surgical or stent therapy.

The major disadvantage of BD is that, although it can immediately dilate both intrinsic and extrinsic lesions, the results are usually not sustainable. Complications are rare, but include chest pain during inflation, bronchospasm, or atelectasis. Other possible complications include airway rupture or laceration by excessive balloon inflation, pneumothorax, pneumomediastinum, or bleeding.

BRACHYTHERAPY

The use of BT has significantly increased as both an adjuvant as well as an alternative radiation option for airway malignancies. There are several advantages of BT over external beam radiation. It can provide a higher dose of radiation to the tumor, minimize the radiation exposure of normal tissue, and dose radiation in a precise location. Because there is a rapid dose "drop-off" with increased distance from the source, there is significantly less injury to the surrounding tissue.

Endobronchial BT is performed by placing the radioactive source through a hollow catheter that is positioned into the endobronchial tree. There is no consensus on the distance prescribed from catheter to tissue, but most authors agree that 1 cm is adequate. The radiation is delivered by an afterloading technique, which involves the placement of a catheter through the bronchoscope to a location that is 2–4 cm distal to the lesion. The catheter is secured, dummy sources are loaded into the catheter, and the radiation dose is calculated. After the position of the catheter is confirmed, the radioactive source replaces the dummy source.

BT can be used by itself or in combination with other endoscopic modalities. Combining laser and BT prolongs symptomatic relief, lessens disease progression, reduces costs, and offers a survival benefit over either modality alone. Aggressive combined therapy with photodynamic therapy (PDT) and BT can improve local tumor control.

The major contraindication of BT is a known fistula to nonbronchial tissue. High-grade obstructions should be debulked prior to BT. It should not be performed in the same endobronchial location for 6 months after the previous full course has been given. The most serious acute complications of BT include fistula formation and massive hemoptysis. Depending on the study reviewed, fistula formation between the airways and other thoracic structures occurred in 1%–8% of patients. The most feared complication is a fistula formation to the mediastinum. Hemoptysis can occur as either an early complication or late complication. Increased risk factors include increased tumor length, anatomical proximity of the pulmonary artery and major vessels to the lesion (right upper lobe, right main stem bronchus, and left upper lobe), recurrent previously irradiated tumor, increased fraction size, and progression of malignant disease. Other acute complications related to the dose include pneumothorax, bronchospasm, bronchial stenosis, and radiation bronchitis.

PHOTODYNAMIC THERAPY

Endobronchial PDT is emerging as an important treatment for lung cancer. There is sufficient evidence that PDT is safe and effective in treating both early- and late-stage malignancy. In advanced disease, its role is palliative. In early-stage disease, its role is of treatment with curative intent.

PDT involves the administration of an intravenous tumor-specific photosensitizing agent that will either be retained in tumor tissue or have selective toxicity for tumor vasculature. These agents remain inactive until they are activated by laser (monochromatic) light administered by bronchoscopy. After activation, a photochemical reaction occurs that produces reactive oxygen singlets; this reaction results in tumor necrosis. Debridement of the necrotic tissue is then performed bronchoscopically 1–2 days after activation. The most commonly used agent is porfimer sodium, which is a hematoporphyrin derivative.

Contraindications to PDT include allergy to porphyrins and porphyria, tracheal–esophageal fistula, or tumor extension into the esophagus or major blood vessels. Complications of PDT include extreme photosensitivity after the procedure, hemoptysis resulting from tumor necrosis, and possible airway edema postprocedure.

The advantage of PDT is its technical ease and safety. There is minimal risk of perforation and minimal residual effects on the normal tissue. The disadvantages of PDT include the need for "clean-up" bronchoscopies, the need to avoid exposure to sunlight for 4–6 weeks, and the slow onset of action. Because of this, PDT is not appropriate for patients with respiratory distress secondary to obstruction.

STENTS

There are a variety of endoscopic interventions available for endoluminal airway obstruction. When obstruction is secondary to extrinsic compression, however, the only sustainable endoscopic procedure available is the placement of a tracheobronchial stent. Stents are essential in maintaining a patent airway in both intrinsic and extrinsic airway obstruction.

The main indication for stent placement is relief of symptoms consistent with airway obstruction from either a malignant or benign obstruction that has failed other medical, surgical, or endoscopic therapies. Table 15.3 describes the indications for stent placement.

In malignancy, stents provide excellent sustainable palliation for progressive symptoms in patients whose conditions have been considered terminal. Improved quality of life and functional benefit have been shown in multiple studies. Increased length of survival has been inferred in a few studies. Stent insertion can be an emergent

Table 15.3. *Indications for tracheobronchial stents*	
Malignant obstruction	**Benign conditions**
Extrinsic compression by tumor or lymphadenopathy	Postintubation tracheal stenosis caused by endotracheal or tracheostomy tubes
Endoluminal proliferation of tumors	Anastomotic stenosis after lung transplantation or surgery
Airway maintenance after debulking	Papillomatosis
Closure of tracheobronchial–esophageal fistula with or without esophageal stent	Tracheobronchomalacia
Airway maintenance before radiation and chemotherapy in large occluding tumors affecting central airways	Tracheobronchial stenosis: idiopathic, Wegener's granulomatosis, relapsing polychondritis, tuberculosis, Sjögren's

Table 15.4. *Comparison of metallic versus silicone stents*

Metallic stents	Silicone stents
Indicated for malignant disease, not indicated in benign disease except as last resource (FDA warning)	Indicated for benign and malignant disease
Inserted with flexible or rigid bronchoscopy	Requires rigid bronchoscopy
Thinner with a greater airway diameter	Thicker with decreased airway diameter
Better able to conform to the airway wall	More difficult to accommodate to an irregular airway narrowing
Fewer secretions problems, especially if the stent is uncovered	Increased secretions
More granulation tissue and mucosal injury	Less mucosal injury and granulation tissue
Difficult to impossible to remove	Easy to remove with rigid bronchoscopy
Difficult to reposition after the stent is in position	Easy to reposition
Migration is common	Migration is common
More expensive	Less expensive
Radiopaque	Not radiopaque
Common brands: Ultraflex® and Alveolus®	Common brands: T tube, Dumon® and Polyflex®

life-saving procedure allowing relief of acute respiratory distress from airway obstruction. It can allow withdrawal from the mechanical ventilator in patients who could not otherwise be extubated.

Over the last 15 years, numerous stents, both metallic and silicone, have evolved from earlier models. Table 15.4 compares characteristics and uses of these two major categories of stents. Metallic stents can be divided into uncovered stainless steel stents (i.e., Gianturco and Palmaz stents) and covered (polyurethane or silicone) stents (i.e., WALLSTENT™, Ultraflex™, and Alveolus™ stents). The covered stents have the benefit of less ingrowth of tissue through the mesh of the stent. The silicone stents are available in both straight and Y shapes.

Currently, there is no ideal stent available that would be appropriate for all types of disorders. Excellent results with stents can be achieved in a majority of patients undergoing the procedure if the patient and the particular stent are selected appropriately.

There are many potential complications that can occur when a tracheobronchial stent is placed. Specific complications can be linked to the particular type of stent that is used.

Migration is one of the most common complications associated with the use of stents. The silicone stents migrate more easily than the metal stents because, as they are deployed, they return to their preformed shape. When metal stents are deployed, they form more to the wall of the airway.

The proliferation of granulation tissue at the proximal and distal ends of the stent is an obstacle that occurs more frequently with metallic stents, and is thought to be secondary to increased irritation to the mucosa by the metallic wire. An improperly sized stent can lead to a higher incidence of granulation tissue formation because of excessive friction against the wall (too small a stent) or to excessive pressure on the bronchial mucosa (too large a stent). The rate and amount of growth of the tissue vary and can range from very little tissue to total obstruction of the stent, requiring either debridement or even removal of the stent. The location of the stent is thought to be associated with the amount of granulation tissue, with the subglottic area being the worst. Obstruction from this proliferative tissue can occur in only a few weeks. Excessive granulation tissue can decrease mucociliary clearance, which can promote infection.

The silicone stents are known for decreasing mucociliary clearance, which can promote the buildup of secretions. This is not as much of a problem in uncovered metallic stents, because the mesh helps to preserve the clearance. Some suggest that chest physiotherapy and inhaled moisturized air and mucolytic can prevent and/or decrease mucous plugging. Bacterial colonization occurs frequently in patients after stenting; however, this does not necessarily lead to clinical infection.

Stent removal can be complicated with metallic wire stents. Placement of metallic stents should be considered permanent as they are difficult (sometimes impossible) to remove after granulation tissue develops through the wire mesh. If they do need to be removed, they must be removed piece by piece with rigid bronchoscopy. For this reason, silicone stents are usually placed for temporary or benign conditions.

CONCLUSION

The discipline of interventional pulmonology is advancing quickly as significant developments occur in both the treatment and diagnostic modalities used for airway and pleural disorders. Considerable progress has been made in this field through education, experience, and new discoveries. This chapter focused primarily on the procedures that are currently the most commonly practiced by interventionalists. These techniques make up the foundation of the field. As the field continues to grow, pulmonary interventionalists will be progressively more responsible for a multitude of new procedures that will incorporate palliation, curative treatments, and early diagnosis of these disorders. This will require the collaborative efforts of pulmonologists, thoracic surgeons, radiologists, radiation oncologists, oncologists, an scientists

working in both industrial and academic settings. Goals of the procedures, technical details, patient selection criteria, complication prevention and management, and alternative treatment strategies must all be integrated when evaluating and performing these procedures.

SUGGESTED READINGS

Bolliger CT, Mathur P, Beamis JF, et al. ERS/ATS statement on interventional pulmonology. European Respiratory Society/American Thoracic Society. *Eur Respir J.* 2002;19(2):356–373.

Cavaliere S, Venuta F, Foccoli P, Toninelli C, La Face B. Endoscopic treatment of malignant airway obstructions in 2,008 patients [published erratum of serious dosage error appears in *Chest.* 1997;111(5):1476]. *Chest.* 1996;110(6):1536–1542.

Chan AL, Yoneda KY, Allen RP, Albertson TE. Advances in the management of endobronchial lung malignancies. *Curr Opin Pulmon Med.* 2003;9(4):301–308.

Coulter TD, Mehta AC. The heat is on: impact of endobronchial electrosurgery on the need for Nd-YAG laser photoresection. *Chest.* 2000;118(2):516–521.

Ernst A, Feller-Kopman D, Becker HD, Mehta AC. Central airway obstruction. *Am J Respir Crit Care Med.* 2004;169(12):1278–1297.

Hautmann H, Gamarra F, Pfeifer KJ, Huber RM. Fiberoptic bronchoscopic balloon dilatation in malignant tracheobronchial disease: indications and results. *Chest.* 2001;120(1):43–49.

Homasson JP. Bronchoscopic cryotherapy. *J Bronchol.* 1995;2:145–149.

Lee P, Kupeli E, Mehta AC. Therapeutic bronchoscopy in lung cancer. Laser therapy, electrocautery, brachytherapy, stents, and photodynamic therapy. *Clin Chest Med.* 2002;23(1):241–256.

Mehrishi S, Ost D. Photodynamic therapy. *J Bronchol.* 2002;9(3):218–222.

Rafanan AL, Mehta AC. Stenting of the tracheobronchial tree. *Radiol Clin North Am.* 2000;38(2):395–408.

Saad CP, Murthy S, Krizmanich G, Mehta AC. Self-expandable metallic airway stents and flexible bronchoscopy: long-term outcomes analysis. *Chest.* 2003;124(5):1993–1999.

Seijo LM, Sterman DH. Interventional pulmonology. *N Engl J Med.* 2001;344(10):740–792.

Turner JF Jr, Wang KP. Endobronchial laser therapy. *Clin Chest Med.* 1999;20(1):107–122.

INDEX